Moving Forward: The Weigh to a Healthier Weight

Moving Forward: The Weigh to a Healthier Weight

✦

A Primer on Healthy Weight Loss without Rigid Dieting

Kathleen T. Baskett, MD

iUniverse, Inc.
New York   Bloomington

Moving Forward: The Weigh to a Healthier Weight
A Primer on Healthy Weight Loss without Rigid Dieting

iUniverse books may be ordered through booksellers or by contacting:

iUniverse
1663 Liberty Drive
Bloomington, IN 47403
www.iuniverse.com
1-800-Authors (1-800-288-4677)

ISBN: 978-0-595-47564-3 (pbk)
ISBN: 978-0-595-71240-3 (cloth)
ISBN: 978-0-595-91831-7 (ebk)

iUniverse Rev Date 11/19/2008
Printed in the United States of America

It has been my privilege and honor to work with many people who have struggled with their weight. I am humbled and honored by their trust in me. I dedicate this book to them.

Contents

Acknowledgments

Writing a book is not something I ever thought I would do. I never considered myself a writer. I like challenges, however, and thought it was time to do something new!

This project has taken a couple of years and has truly been a journey for me. I would like to thank the editorial staff at iUniverse, especially Sarah Disbrow. Sarah was patient and encouraging, and she prodded me to move forward at times of discouragement.

I wish to thank the staff at the St. Vincent Healthcare Weight Management Clinic. We have a strong team of caring professionals, and their comments and input have been invaluable.

A special thanks to my assistant in Missoula, Summer Rose, who always found a few extra hours in my schedule for me to work on my book. She handled matters at the office smoothly and efficiently while I had to be away.

Of course, this book could not have been written without my patients. I have learned much from them and am so grateful that they have allowed me to be a part of their lives.

Last, but not least, I wish to acknowledge and thank my husband and best friend, Mark Bassingthwaighte. He is my best critic—honest and kind. He has given me the encouragement and the freedom to pursue my dreams!

1

Diets Don't Work!

There are so many diet books that promise a quick and easy way to lose weight. They also imply that if you follow their plan, you will lose weight, look beautiful, and be happy forever.

Well, it's clear that, in the long run, diets don't work! Many dieters are able to lose weight, but very few are successful in keeping it off. There is no long-term data to suggest that people who go on a diet *stay* on that diet. Most diets involve denial and restriction and often, in the long run, result in hunger and cravings for "forbidden foods." In addition, restrictive diets are not healthy over the long term because of the exclusion of important foods that provide us with needed vitamins, minerals, protein, and, yes, even fats (Freedman, King, and Kennedy 2001). Thus, a diet is something you will stop. It is a temporary solution to a lifelong issue.

What I want to share with you in this book is a healthier way—a way to lose weight slowly and steadily, maintain your new weight, and have a healthier relationship with food. This will take work and commitment on your part—in reality, there is no quick fix. However, shedding pounds and maintaining a healthy weight is not a mysterious process. Others have done it. You can, too!

Bariatric medicine deals with the prevention, treatment, and control of obesity and its associated diseases. A bariatric physician uses a combination of customized eating and exercise plans, educates and motivates with regards to lifestyle change, and, if necessary, prescribes medication to help a patient achieve and maintain a healthy weight.

As a bariatric physician, I have worked with thousands of people struggling with weight issues. Some of these people need to lose fifteen pounds, and others need to lose 200 or more pounds. Each person has an individual story and struggles. Unfortunately, some suffered discrimination from society and even from the medical profession.

Because obesity is a visible condition that one cannot hide, overweight people are often subjected to the comments, judgment, and scorn of those who do not struggle with their weight. I have encountered patients who do not want to go outside during the day to do their walking. They prefer to do it at night, when people "will not see me." They share stories of how they have been walking along and feeling good about their progress, only to have someone in a passing car yell out obscenities and remarks about their size.

More than one of my patients has told me, "There isn't a day that goes by that somebody doesn't remind me that I'm fat." They are often asked, "When are you going to lose some weight?" Conversely, but just as distressingly, many of my overweight patients have related how they are often *not* noticed. One of my patients, Eileen (patient names have been changed to protect their identities), shared with me that when she was of a larger size and would take her car in to the dealer for service, none of the staff would acknowledge her. She would have to ask repeatedly for help. After losing a hundred pounds, she was astounded by how much more frequently people noticed her, paid attention to her, and treated her courteously.

Physicians will often tell their overweight patients, "Just eat less and exercise more," or, even more insensitively, "Come back to see me after you lose some weight."

All of this leads to the feelings of shame and guilt that many overweight people struggle with. Patients will often tell me that they are "bad" because they cannot control their eating and their weight.

Of course, your eating and activity are very important. However, weight regulation involves multiple interacting factors, and it is a complex and delicately balanced process. Some of these factors are beyond your control—I'll review some of these in chapter 5—and so we should not make moral judgments about the character of someone who is overweight. Losing weight and keeping it off is not an easy task. It is a challenging and ongoing one. At the same time, it *is* doable. You may not be the next Victoria's Secret or *GQ* model, but you *can* reach a healthier weight—one that will improve your health and the quality of your life.

Many people who walk through my office door are actually experts at dieting. They have tried just about every diet out there: Atkins, South Beach, SlimFast, The Zone, Cabbage Soup—you name it. They have read the best-selling diet books, followed the latest diet craze, and purchased diet pills and other aids. Lots of these people have lost weight. However, they have not been able to maintain their new weight after dieting. They have regained their lost weight, and then some. They have lost healthy, lean muscle mass, added more fat mass to their bodies, and wreaked havoc on their metabolisms. They are discouraged, and they are tired of the roller coaster. They cannot manage their weight because they have not developed the skills to do so.

My goal in this book is to teach you these skills and to help you develop the habits that will lead to healthy and successful weight management.

I believe that it is important for you to understand the implications of carrying around too much weight, which I will discuss in chapter 3. Of course, people are concerned about their outward appearance, but I want you to have an understanding of the effects of too much adipose tissue (fat) on the body and its systems. Then, I want you to decide what to do about it.

According to the Centers for Disease Control (CDC), obesity is now the second leading cause of preventable death in this country because of its significant health-related issues (Mokdad, Marks, and Stroup 2000, 1238–1245). Reaching a healthier weight will offer you the potential for a healthier and improved quality of life.

If you choose to embark on a weight-loss program, make sure that this is something that *you* want to do and that you are ready to do. Losing weight to please your spouse or another family member or friend usually does not result in long-term weight loss, because you are not invested in or committed to the process. Likewise, although you may know that you need to lose weight and want to do so, it has to be the right time for you. If you have a more-than-full-time career, a busy family, and multiple community commitments, where is the time to prioritize yourself and your health? Chapter 8 reviews this topic, and it can help you make the right decision—for you.

One of the reasons why people do not reach a healthy weight is that they are not ready to make a commitment to themselves. When the first stumbling block comes along, they feel overwhelmed and give up. We will talk about being ready and about how to determine whether this is the right time for you to work on weight loss. Also, because I am not providing you with a diet, there will be no strict regime for you to abandon—no detailed eating plan for you to quit.

You might be thinking, "Not again—I just can't fail again!" In order to make failure less likely, I will be challenging you to try something new—something that makes common sense.

Remember, this is not a diet book. This book will show you how to lose weight in a healthy way. We will tackle the issue step by step and divide your overall weight-loss goal into small segments.

Chapter 4 will offer you the tools to get started on your weight-loss journey and discuss how you can maintain your new weight indefinitely. Chapter 5 will discuss what is involved in weight regulation and explain why you weigh what you do. Other chapters will talk about challenging situations like family gatherings and restaurant outings, and how you can still lose weight while living life.

I cannot offer you a quick and easy fix, but I *can* help you through this learning process. The Greek word for diet is *diaita,* which means "manner of living." You are going to learn how to develop a healthy way of living that will help you reach your goal of a healthier weight. *You can do this.*

The majority of patients with whom I work have been successful in achieving a healthier weight, but it is an ongoing challenge for them to *maintain* that new weight. After weight loss, one's fat cells remain, waiting to be refilled (picture a collapsed balloon with the potential to be filled with air). Once you have a weight issue, you tend to always have a weight issue. It does not simply disappear with the pounds you have lost. Those people who continue with their new habits have the greatest chance of staying at their new weight. Although it can be daunting to deal with eating problems and weight issues, the process can be immensely rewarding. I look forward to sharing this journey with you.

I have worked in the field of bariatric medicine for many years. People will often ask me why I have chosen to do so. My undergraduate studies were in health science and education, and I have always had an interest in nutrition and fitness. While practicing primary care medicine, I encountered many patients struggling with and seeking help for weight and eating issues. Thus, it seemed to be a natural progression for me to delve into the area of bariatric medicine.

For me, there is much joy and reward knowing that I can help a person deal with an ongoing and chronic issue, and that I can guide that person toward making positive lifestyle changes. The process of growth and improved health in an individual is an honor to share. My hope is that this book will lead you to a better understanding of how complex weight regulation is and that you will develop the knowledge and skills to reach and maintain a healthier weight. I want you to be proud of yourself and your body, knowing that each of us naturally comes in a different shape and size.

I think that most of us hope to make a difference in this life. I hope that I have done so, for my patients and for you.

QUESTIONS TO ASK YOURSELF

1. Do I need to lose weight?

2. What diets have I tried in the past?

3. What is the largest amount of weight I have ever lost?

4. What has been my highest weight as an adult?

5. What has been my lowest weight as an adult?

6. What weight have I been able to maintain, as an adult, for at least eighteen months?

MOVING FORWARD

1. Diets do not work.

2. It is time to develop healthy habits to help you reach a healthier weight.

3. Reaching a healthier weight is a process, not a race.

2

Am I Overweight? Could I Really Be Obese?

Before we go any further, let's define the term *obesity*. Nobody likes to think of themselves as being overweight, let alone obese. It's one thing to carry an extra ten or fifteen pounds, but what about an extra twenty to thirty pounds, or even much more? Interestingly, in 2007, the National Consumer League (NCL) commissioned Harris Interactive to conduct an online survey of adult Americans on issues related to weight and obesity. The results were as follows (National Consumer League Obesity Survey 2007):

U.S. adults were more likely to refer to themselves as "overweight" rather than "obese."

They consistently identified themselves as being less severely overweight than they actually were.

Fifty-two percent of respondents identified themselves as being overweight.

Twelve percent of respondents identified themselves as being obese.

Based on actual BMI calculations, 35 percent of respondents were overweight and 34 percent were obese.

THE BODY MASS INDEX (BMI)

Obviously, there is a disconnect between the way people perceive their weight and their actual weight category based on the BMI. What is the BMI? The body mass index, or BMI, is a measure of the distribution of your weight over your body frame. This number is an objective and fairly accurate indicator of one's general health. This number can indicate how you are doing in the weight department and whether or not you may want to consider losing a few or more pounds.

Calculate your BMI by converting your weight from pounds to kilograms and then dividing by your height in meters squared:

Weight = # pounds x 0.45

Height = (# inches x 0.025) squared

Example: 220 pounds and five feet four inches in height.

220 x 0.45 = 99
64 inches x 0.025 = 1.6

1.6 X 1.6 = 2.56
99 divided by 2.56 = 38.6

Thus, the BMI is 38.6 and is consistent with obesity.

Calculate your own BMI here:

Your weight _____ x 0.45 (A)

Your height _____ x 0.025 then squared (B)

Weight figure A _____ divided by height figure B _____ = _____: your personal BMI calculation.

You can also reference the BMI table below for a general BMI number.

Body Mass Index Chart

Weight (lb)

Height (ft)	120	130	140	150	160	170	180	190	200	210	220	230	240	250	260	270	280	290	300	320	340	360	380	400
60	23	25	27	29	31	33	35	37	39	41	43	45	47	49	51	53	55	57	59	63	66	70	74	78
62	22	24	26	27	29	31	33	35	37	38	40	42	44	46	48	49	51	53	55	59	62	66	70	73
64	21	22	24	26	28	29	31	33	34	36	38	40	41	43	45	46	48	50	52	55	58	62	65	69
66	19	21	23	24	26	27	29	31	32	34	36	37	39	40	42	44	45	47	49	52	55	58	61	65
68	18	20	21	23	24	26	27	29	30	32	34	35	37	38	40	41	43	44	46	48	52	55	58	61
70	17	19	20	22	23	24	26	27	29	30	32	33	35	36	37	39	40	42	43	46	49	52	55	57
72	16	18	19	20	22	23	24	26	27	29	30	31	33	34	35	37	38	39	41	43	46	49	52	54
74	15	17	18	19	21	22	23	24	26	27	28	30	31	32	33	35	36	37	39	41	44	46	49	51
76	15	16	17	18	20	21	22	23	24	26	27	28	29	30	32	33	34	35	37	40	41	44	46	49

Slide Source:
www.obesityonline.org

Figure 1
Body Mass Index Chart

A BMI greater than twenty-five is consistent with being overweight. A BMI of thirty or greater is consistent with obesity. A BMI between twenty-seven and thirty, especially when associated with other medical conditions (high blood pressure, diabetes, polycystic ovarian disease (PCOS), and sleep apnea, to name a few), is of concern.

Realize that these are not arbitrary numbers, but indicators of when many of the medical consequences of having too much adipose (fat) tissue begin to develop. When the BMI reaches thirty and above, the risk for developing high blood pressure, coronary artery disease, sleep apnea, type 2 (adult onset) diabetes, high cholesterol, and some types of cancers increases dramatically.

BMI	Health Risk Based on BMI Alone	Risk Based on BMI with Associated Diseases
< 25	Minimal	Low
25–27	Low	Moderate
27–30	Moderate	High
30–35	High	Very High
35–40	Very High	Extremely High
> 40	Extremely High	Extremely High

Your Waist-Hip Ratio (WHR)

In addition to the BMI, we have to consider some other measurements. A BMI alone is not indicative of being overweight. For example, a heavily muscled man or a pregnant woman would have a high BMI, but neither person would be obese. Muscle weighs more than fat, so people who are densely muscular will weigh more, yet not be obese. A pregnant woman is heavier for even more obvious reasons, but is likely perfectly healthy.

The Waist-Hip Ratio (WHR) is a more accurate individual indicator of cardiovascular disease. It is useful in assessing body-fat distribution, as upper-body or abdominal obesity is known to increase health risk. The WHR is calculated by dividing the waist measurement by the hip measurement.

For example, a woman with a waist measurement of 36" and a hip measurement of 38" would calculate her WHR like this: 36 divided by 38 equals 0.947.

> Calculate your WHR here:
> Waist measurement _____
> Hip measurement _____
> Waist divided by hip measurement = _____. This is your WHR.

Men with a WHR over 1.0 and women over 0.85 are considered at high risk for cardiovascular disease. For measurement purposes, the waist lies midway between the lowest rib bone and the top of the hip bone. A waist measurement of thirty-five inches or greater in women or forty inches or greater in men is consistent with too much adipose tissue. Abdominal (or "visceral") fat has negative health implications. There is a 97 percent correlation between a higher waist measurement and the development of diabetes and heart disease. Excessive visceral fat is also associated with the development of colon and breast cancers (European Heart Journal Supplement 2005).

It is interesting to note that someone at a "normal" weight may have an excess of this visceral fat, and therefore have an increased risk of health problems. Studies have shown that people who are thinner, yet have a history of extreme dieting, often have more of this visceral fat. Each time they lose weight and then regain the lost weight, more fat is deposited internally in the abdominal area.

So, if your BMI is greater than twenty-seven and your waistline has expanded, you may want to consider making some changes in your life to reach a healthier weight.

Case Study: Steve

"I'm not that overweight."

Steve came to see me at the urging of his orthopedic physician. Steve had been having ongoing back and knee problems for years. Now, at the age of fifty, he was facing the possibility of a knee replacement. Since Steve was still relatively young, his surgeon was hesitant to perform the surgery and explained that Steve's weight might be contributing to his knee problems.

Steve was a bit disbelieving, stating that "I know I carry a few extra pounds, but I am not that overweight .... I just want to get this surgery done and move on with my life." Steve did not even know just how much he weighed. He ate "what I want," and he did have a physically active job as a foreman on a construction crew. He was married and the father of four and did not have much time for many extra activities in his life.

Steve was on two high blood pressure medications and CPAP for his sleep apnea. His weight was 260 pounds, and he was 5'8" in height. His waist measurement was 42". Steve's BMI was 40, which is consistent with morbid obesity. Steve was shocked. He never thought of himself as "that heavy."

I explained to Steve that his high blood pressure and sleep apnea, as well as his degenerative joint issues, were in large part related to his excessive weight. He was open to beginning a structured weight-loss program and agreed to follow up with me next week.

QUESTIONS TO ASK YOURSELF

1. Do I think I am overweight?

2. What is my BMI?

3. What is my WHR?

MOVING FORWARD

1. The BMI refers to the distribution of your weight over your body frame.

2. A BMI of thirty or greater is associated with obesity.

3. As the BMI increases, so does the risk for developing many diseases.

4. A waist measurement of greater than thirty-five for women or forty for men is consistent with abdominal obesity.

5. Know your BMI and WHR.

3

What's Wrong with Carrying a Little Extra Weight?

○ ○

More people die in the United States of too much food than of too little.

—John Kenneth Galbraith

So, just what is the big deal about being a little (or a lot) overweight? Isn't it normal to weigh more as you age? Maybe. Often, as people get older, they become busy with raising a family and building their careers. Little time is left for exercise or even healthy eating. There is a gradual climb in weight year by year. Couple this with a slowing of metabolism and the loss of lean muscle mass, and even more weight gain can occur. Yet, this does not always have to be the case.

Isn't it true that, in some cultures, excessive weight was valued as a sign of prosperity? Perhaps so, but something being or having been a cultural tradition doesn't necessarily make it a healthy practice. In any case, in the U.S. today, extra weight tends not to carry any such positive connotations.

In our country, over 66 percent of the population is overweight or obese.

Overweight is defined as the state of having a BMI of 25–29.9. This correlates with being up to thirty pounds over your healthy weight. For example, a woman who is 5'4" tall and weighs 160 pounds has a BMI of 28.1. She would be considered overweight.

Obesity is defined as the state of having a BMI of thirty or greater. This correlates with *being more than* thirty pounds over your healthy weight. For example, a man who is 5'10" and weighs 210 pounds has a BMI of 31.5. He would be considered obese.

Morbid obesity is defined as the state of having a BMI of forty or greater. This correlates with being one hundred pounds or more over your healthy weight. For example, a woman who is 5'4" and weighs 240 pounds has a BMI of 42.1. This meets the medical definition of morbid obesity.

Obesity is now the second leading cause of preventable death, behind smoking. But obesity is quickly catching up. It has been determined that 300,000 to 500,000 people die each year from the effects of poor diet and inactivity (Flegal, Carroll, Ogden, and Johnson 2002, 1723–1727). We know that 300,000 people per year do actually die as a direct result of obesity (Allison, Fontaine, Manson, Stevens, and Van Itallie 1999, 1530–1538), and research has shown that the effects of obesity are similar to those of twenty years of aging (Sturm 2002). Clearly, obesity is a real health problem in our country. Many of our chronic diseases are the result of being overweight and leading a sedentary lifestyle. These chronic diseases include:

Heart disease
Diabetes mellitus type 2
Sleep apnea
Degenerative joint disease
Cancer
High blood pressure
Elevated cholesterol
Polycystic Ovarian Syndrome (PCOS)

Pseudotumor cerebri and infertility are other medical conditions associated with obesity. Pseudotumor cerebri is a condition most commonly seen in women between the ages of twenty and fifty. An actual tumor is not present, but the symptoms can mimic those of a brain tumor. It is due to increased pressure of fluid in the brain, and symptoms can include nausea, vomiting, headache, and vision problems.

Obese people have more work-related injuries, miss more days of work, and have a generally poorer quality of life than their nonobese neighbors. Morbid obesity is a complex and chronic disease that affects the entire body and its internal organs. Although it cannot be cured, it can be controlled.

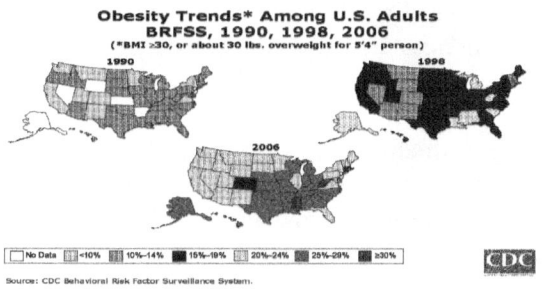

Figure 4
Obesity Trends Among U.S. Adults

In addition, over 25 percent of our children and adolescents are obese (Collins et al. 2007, 147–152). Many of the typical "adult" diseases, such as diabetes, high cholesterol, high blood pressure, and heart disease—in other words, diseases related to lifestyle—are now being seen in these overweight children and teens. Again, this is due to the fact that these young people are carrying around too much weight, usually due to poor food choices and an inactive lifestyle.

The figure above depicts the increasing occurrence of obesity in our society. In 1990, among states that participated in the Behavioral Risk Factor Surveillance System, ten had a prevalence of obesity under 10 percent. No states had an occurrence of obesity equal to or greater than 15 percent.

By 1998, no state had a prevalence of obesity under 10 percent. Seven states had a prevalence of obesity between 20 and 24 percent. No state had a prevalence equal to or greater than 25 percent.

In 2006, only four states had a prevalence of obesity under 20 percent. Twenty-two states had a prevalence equal to or greater than 25 percent, and two of these states (Mississippi and West Virginia) had a prevalence of obesity equal to or greater than 30 percent.

Examples of these statistics walk through the doors of my office each day. After many years of working with overweight and obese people, I know that achieving a healthy weight is not as simple as eating less and exercising more. Of course, these things are important, and yet millions of people have dieted only to regain any weight lost, and then some. People have suffered incredible anxiety, agony, and shame over their body size and their failed attempts to reach their "ideal" weight. People are susceptible to the latest diet fad or gimmick that promises fast weight loss. We live in a fast-paced society and like things to change at the touch of a computer key. One often has the feeling that weight gain happened "overnight," and therefore, this weight should be lost just as quickly. It doesn't work that way. Why you weigh what you do is very complicated, and certain factors are beyond your control. We will talk about some of these factors in the next chapter. Remember, diets do not work, and not all women are meant to be a size six—let alone a size zero! All men do not need to have a 32" or 34" waist.

What *is* important, though, is that you achieve and maintain a healthy weight for *you*—one at which you have a lower risk for life-threatening disease and are able to be physically active and keep up with the demands of your daily life. Technically, your weight may not reach the "ideal" number found on a chart. It doesn't have to. Research has shown that if a person can lose even 5 to 10 percent of his starting body weight, there will be improvement in health and a reduction in risk factors (Archives Internal Medicine 2000, World Health Organization 1998).

So, if you can lose twenty to thirty pounds and maintain that loss, you will be a healthier and fitter person. You will notice the difference in your body if you lose this amount of weight. You will be able to breathe more easily. You will be able to move more easily. You will be able to get down on the floor to play with your children or grandchildren. You will not need that seat-belt extender. Your blood-sugar levels and blood pressure will improve. You might be able to discontinue some of your medications. Allow these possibilities to motivate you and reinforce your will to succeed!

Case Study: Louise

"I really want to have a baby."

Louise was a thirty-two-year-old woman who had been married for seven years and had not been able to have a baby. She and her husband had been evaluated by her obstetrician, and their test results were all within normal limits. The doctor was concerned that her weight was the reason behind her infertility. Louise came to see me for help in losing weight.

Louise told me that she had struggled with her weight for most of her life. She currently was at her highest weight, and she wanted to do "whatever it took" to lose weight and get healthier, because she so wanted to have a baby.

Louise weighed 220 pounds, and she was 5'4" tall. Her BMI was thirty-eight. Tests revealed that she had a HgbA1C (test for diabetes) of 7.5, which is positive for diabetes type 2, and her blood pressure was 140/90. Louise's triglycerides were also high at 422. So, not only was Louise dealing with infertility, she also had high blood pressure, diabetes, and high triglycerides.

Over the period of a year, I was able to work with Louise, and she lost thirty pounds. This 15 percent reduction of her initial body weight resulted in the resolution of her diabetes and high blood pressure. Her triglycerides normalized to 150. Louise was a bit disappointed that she couldn't seem to lose more weight, but she was thrilled with the improvement in her health.

Unfortunately, I lost contact with Louise the following year, as she and her husband moved to another state. However, about a year later, I received a note from her, with a family picture. She wrote that she had worked hard to maintain her weight and had finally become pregnant. She had given birth to a beautiful girl the month before and had sent me a picture of the three of them!

QUESTIONS TO ASK YOURSELF

1. What medical conditions am I dealing with?

2. What medications do I take?

3. What is 5 percent of my current weight?

4. What is 10 percent of my current weight?

5. Do I think I can lose and keep off 5 to 10 percent of my current weight?

MOVING FORWARD

1. The prevalence of obesity in the United States is steadily increasing.

2. Many illnesses are associated with obesity. These include diabetes type 2, high blood pressure, high cholesterol, sleep apnea, and cancer.

3. Even a 5 to 10 percent maintained weight loss can greatly improve your health.

4

How Do I Lose Weight?

Habit is habit and not to be flung out of the window by any man,
but coaxed downstairs, a step at a time.

—Mark Twain

Congratulations! You have made the decision to take the initiative to lose weight and improve your health, so let's move forward. Remember, you are *not* going to be on a diet. A diet is something that has an end—it is something that one eventually discontinues. You, on the other hand, are going to develop some healthy, long-term habits that will allow you to lose weight and, more importantly, keep it off. Believe it or not, this will not be painful. *Slow and steady* will be your motto.

Personally, I think that a medically supervised weight-loss program in conjunction with lifestyle change will offer you the greatest opportunity for success. Find a medical professional who has expertise in the area of bariatric medicine. This person should be knowledgeable, supportive, and caring. Working with someone who tells you to close your mouth, eat less, and exercise more will most likely not be helpful. A listing of bariatric physicians can be found on the Web site of the American Society of Bariatric Physicians (ASBP). (Please see the Reader Resource section of this book.)

When I see a patient for weight loss, I take complete medical and weight histories. I also assess his or her readiness. If the patient is ready to proceed, I conduct a more detailed evaluation consisting of a physical examination, comprehensive laboratory studies, measurement of body composition, evaluation of resting metabolic rate (RMR), and an electrocardiogram (ECG).

I then review the results of all this with my patient and develop an individualized eating plan. *Individualized* is the key word here. There is no one-size-fits-all weight-loss program. What works for one person will not necessarily work for another. Again, I stress that this is *not* meant to be a diet, but the beginning of a series of lifestyle changes. You will make decisions and choices about your life and what you are able and willing to modify. This is a process that will take time and work, but one that is most doable and not complicated. We will talk about the importance of knowing your resting metabolic rate, review what to eat and when, and use food records, increased activity, and medication and/or surgery to help you reach your goals.

RMR

I don't think I even have a metabolism.

—Patient

In order for you to achieve a healthy weight, you need to identify your target calorie intake goal. This is best achieved by measuring your RMR (resting metabolic rate). Each person has a unique RMR—and yes, everybody *does* have a metabolism! Two people can be of the same gender, height, and weight, yet their RMR can vary by as much as 900 points. Knowing your RMR can help you determine how many calories you should consume daily in order to lose weight. The Body Gem/Med Gem and the REEVUE are two calorimeters now available in the clinical setting that are used to accurately measure one's RMR. The calorimeter will provide a more accurate measurement of a person's metabolism, as it accounts for the individual differences between people, which standardized formulas do not.

However, if you do not have the option of having your RMR measured, you can calculate, in general, the calories your body needs to function with the following formula:

1. Take your weight in pounds and convert it to kilograms by dividing it by 2.2

2. Take your height in inches and convert it to centimeters by multiplying it by 2.54

3. Insert these numbers and your age into the following equation:

10 × weight (kg) + 6.25 x height (cm) – 5 * (your age) – 161 = RMR

This result will give you an estimate of your RMR. Here is an example:

225 pounds divided by 2.2 = 102 kilograms

63 inches in height multiplied by 2.54 = 160 centimeters

Age = 38

Therefore:

(10 × 102) + (6.25 × 160) – (5 × 38) – 161

10 × 102 = 1020   6.25 × 160 = 1000   5 × 38 = 190

1020 + 1000 = 2020

2020 – 190 = 1830

1830 – 161 = 1669

1669 = RMR

Calculate Your RMR:

Weight in pounds divided by 2.2 = Weight(kg) = A
Height in inches multiplied by 2.54 = Height(cm) = B
Age multiplied by 5 = _____ = C

A × 10 = _____ = D
B × 6.25 = _____ = E

D + E = _____ minus C = _____ minus 161 = _____ = RMR

This final figure is your RMR.

Subtract 200 to 400 from your RMR number. This is your *net calorie goal* for one day. Therefore, in the above example:

1669 – 400 = **1269 = Net Calorie Goal for the day**

Your net calorie goal is the number of calories taken in minus the number of calories expended. Achieving this calorie goal, with the help of consistent and intentional activity, will result in a slow and steady weight loss. For example, if you took in 1669 calories for the day and walked four miles that day (burning 400 calories), your net calorie intake for the day would be 1269. This will result in weight loss.

To simplify even further, women might try a 1400-calorie-per-day eating plan, and men might try an 1800-calorie-per-day eating plan. If you are losing weight too quickly (more than two or three pounds per week), give yourself more calories. If you aren't losing weight at all, you may need to cut back your caloric intake.

These calculations assume that your exercise is adequate. If your eating plan allows you 1400 calories per day, what is the best way to do this? Incorporate a variety of foods throughout the day. If you choose to spend 200 calories on cookies, you then have 1200 calories left for other foods. Make healthy and nutritious choices, but do not deny yourself. You are not "bad" for having a dish of ice cream each evening. If this is important to you, make it a part of your eating plan and allow for the calories from that scoop of ice cream. Rigid eating and a narrow variety of foods will ultimately lead to overeating and possibly binging.

For most people, weight gain is gradual. You truly did not go to bed one night wearing a size eight and wake up the next morning barely fitting into a size fourteen. Because the weight gain has occurred over a period of time, it is desirable to have a slow, steady weight loss. By losing the weight slowly, you will maintain your lean muscle mass and keep your metabolism running smoothly. The goal is to change your habits so that when a healthy weight is reached, it can be maintained. Record keeping is one of the skills that will help you to do this.

FOOD RECORDS

For the two out of three Americans who do not smoke and drink excessively, one personal choice seems to influence long-term health more than any other—what we eat.

—Surgeon General's report on nutrition, 1988

Due to increases in portion sizes, we have lost perspective on what a true serving size is, and so many of us take in more food than we realize. In fact, people tend to underestimate their intake by as much as 25 to 30 percent, which can account for a lot of additional calories. These additional calories add up and result in excess pounds. Therefore, keeping a food diary is an invaluable tool (Lichtman et al. 1992, 1893–1898).

Food records help you to see just what you are taking in, and how much. In addition to recording the foods you eat, it is helpful to jot down some notes as to how you feel emotionally that day, what your stressors are, and your level of hunger. By doing this, you will increase your awareness of what you are eating and whether or not you are truly hungry. You will also be able to see the relationship between increased anxiety, boredom, or loneliness and the types and quantities of foods you eat. This increased awareness can give you more control and the ability to make the necessary changes to lose weight.

For example, you look over your records for the past few days and realize that you have been coming home after some very stressful days at work and eating half a bag of chips and drinking two gin and tonics while preparing dinner. Before dinner on each of those days, you had already taken in 1,200 calories. You did this almost without thinking about it or being aware of those extra calories. But now, after examining your diary, you *are* aware, and you can make some decisions about how to handle the stress differently, without mindless eating.

It's best to record your foods at the time you eat them or right after. After a busy day, most people can't recall everything they had to eat—exactly how many chips with lunch or how many ounces of milk on their morning cereal. It's even more difficult to remember these things the next day or at the end of the week!

In addition to recording your food and beverages, it's also important to calculate the calorie content of each item. The only way to determine the calorie content of a food is to calculate the quantity of that food. So, when at home, pull out your measuring cups, tablespoons, teaspoons, and food scale. The basic equations still apply:

CALORIES IN = CALORIES OUT = MAINTENANCE

CALORIES IN > CALORIES OUT = WEIGHT GAIN

CALORIES IN < CALORIES OUT = WEIGHT LOSS

Figure 5
Calorie Intake Effects

About twenty years ago, some food companies began to "supersize" their portions. Bagels and muffins got bigger, as did the standard size of a soft drink. Restaurants began using larger plates and putting more food on them. Studies have shown that many of us rely on visual clues to help us determine when we are full (Wansink 2006). In other words, if our plate still has food on it, we think that we must still be hungry, and we will eat until the plate is clean.

Become familiar with what four ounces of chicken looks like and what one cup of mashed potatoes looks like. The better you are at measuring your foods and calculating calories, the better you will be able to estimate what a true serving size is when you are eating out. The following table will give you some guidelines to help you more accurately estimate serving sizes.

ONE SERVING OF	IS ABOUT THE SIZE OF
Raw vegetables	Fist
Cooked vegetables	Palm of hand
Pasta	One ice cream scoop
Meat	Deck of cards
Grilled fish	Checkbook
2 Tbsp. butter, cream cheese, peanut butter	Thumb (joint to tip)
Snacks (pretzels, chips)	Handful
Apple	Baseball
Potato	Computer mouse
Bagel (1/2)	Hockey puck
Pancake	Compact disc
Steamed rice	Cupcake wrapper
Cheese	Pair of dice

Take a look at the following sample food and activity records. Note that all foods are recorded, along with their portion sizes and calorie counts. Also recorded are the step counts from the person's pedometer. More information about pedometers will follow in the section on exercise.

Food Record #1 contains many high-fat, high-calorie foods eaten by a person who is sedentary. The total calorie intake for this person for the day is 5250 calories. This person put 3000 steps on his pedometer, resulting in 150 exercise calories burned for the day (**2000 steps is equivalent to one mile. Walking one mile burns about 100 calories).** Thus, the person's net calorie intake for the day is 5100 calories (total calorie intake minus exercise calories). This is an excessive amount, one that inevitably leads to weight gain.

Food Record #2 shows how a few changes can lead to a significantly lower calorie intake. Couple this with a little more movement, and the net intake for the day is 1765 calories. This is much more conducive to reaching a healthier weight, and it is accomplished without denying oneself.

Table 2— Sample Food Record *

Food Record #1		Calories Food	Calories Exercise	Grams Protein
BREAKFAST	Caffe Mocha, 16 oz	660		13 g
SNACK	Krispy Kreme donuts, 2 glazed	410		
LUNCH	McDonald's Quarter Pounder with cheese	510		29 g
	Large Fries	570		6 g
	Strawberry Milkshake, 32 oz	1110		25 g
SNACK	KitKat bar, large	290		
DINNER	Pepperoni pizza, 3 slices	780		36 g
	Pepsi, 2 cans	300		
EVENING SNACK	Ben & Jerry's ice cream, Everything But The ... – ½ pint	620		10 g
Pedometer	3000 Steps		150	
	TOTAL	5250	150	119 g
	NET CALORIES	5100		

*   (Net calories = Total calories in – Exercise calories)

Table 3—Sample Food Record with Modifications *

Food Record #2		Calories Food	Calories Exercise	Protein Grams
BREAKFAST	Yogurt – ½ cup	110		5 g
	Granola bar	120		2g
SNACK	Nonfat latte, 16 oz	100		13 g
LUNCH	Subway sandwich, 6″ turkey breast	280		17 g
	Apple	70		
	Chips Ahoy snack pack cookies	100		
	Bottled water	0		
SNACK	Peanuts, 2 oz	320		14 g
	Pepsi, 12 oz	150		
DINNER	Pepperoni pizza, 2 slices	520		24 g
	Carrot & celery sticks, 1 cup each	35		
	Water	0		
EVENING SNACK	Ben & Jerry's ice cream, Everything But The ... – ½ cup	310		5 g
Pedometer	5000 steps		250	
	TOTAL	2015	250	80 g
	NET CALORIES	1765		

*   (Net calories = Total calories in – Exercise calories)

Record #3 is that of a person needing to take in 1400 calories per day to lose weight. This person, however, exceeded that amount by 455 calories. Record #4 shows how a few changes here and there, both with food intake and activity output, will get that person to the desired caloric balance for the day.

Table 4—Sample Food Record—Over Calorie Budget *

Food Record #3		Calories Food	Calories Exercise	Grams Protein
BREAKFAST	Yogurt, 1 cup	220		10 g
	Banana, medium	105		
	½ bagel, 2 oz	150		
	Cream cheese, 1 oz	80		
	Coffee, black	0		
SNACK	Almonds, 1 oz	170		4 g
LUNCH	Fruit/Walnut salad, McDonald's	210		4 g
	McDonald's cheeseburger	310		15 g
	Bottled water	0		
SNACK	Protein shake	110		15 g
DINNER	Grilled halibut, 4 oz	200		28 g
	Salad w/ Italian dressing, 1 oz	150		
	Steamed green beans, 1 cup	30		
	Brown rice, 1 cup	220		
	White wine, 8 oz	200		
Pedometer	6000 steps		300	
	TOTAL	2155	300	76 g
	NET CALORIES	1855		

*   (Net calories = Total calories in – Exercise calories)

Table 5— Sample Food Record with Modifications *

Food Record #4		Calories Food	Calories Exercise	Grams Protein
BREAKFAST	Yogurt, 1 cup	220		10 g
	Banana, medium	105		
	Coffee, black	<1		
SNACK	Almonds, 1 oz	170		4 g
LUNCH	Fruit/Walnut salad	210		4 g
	McDonald's cheeseburger	310		15 g
	Bottled water	0		
SNACK	Protein shake	110		15 g
DINNER	Grilled halibut , 4 oz	200		28 g
	Mixed lettuce salad w/ Italian dressing, 1 oz	150		
	Steamed green beans , 1 cup	30		
	Brown rice, ½ cup	110		
	White wine, 4 oz	100		
Pedometer	8000 steps		400	
	TOTAL	1715	400	76 g
	NET CALORIES	1315		

*   (Net calories = Total calories in – Exercise calories)

You may want to think of your record keeping as similar to the way you keep records for your checking account. You have a budget for the day (e.g., 1500 calories). Food (calorie) intake is analogous to a withdrawal. Activity is a deposit. The more active you are, the more you can eat and still lose weight! I have encountered many people who really don't like to exercise, but they do so regularly in order to enjoy their food—and a lot of it!

Remember, this isn't about denial. You can eat foods you enjoy and drink beverages that you like. However, to reach a healthy weight, you need to take control, make smart choices, adjust your portion sizes, and increase your activity. Small changes over time can result in a positive outcome. For example, if you cut out one sugary soft drink per day and the rest of your diet remained the same, you would lose about twelve pounds in a year. Likewise, if you walked one extra mile per day, you would burn an extra 100 calories per day, which would add up to a ten-pound weight loss in one year.

Granted, keeping a food record can be tedious. If, after a while, you find it too difficult to maintain, consider keeping the record for two days a week and one weekend a month. On these days, you would commit to weighing, measuring, and recording your foods. This will help you to double-check yourself and determine if your guesstimates have been accurate. For those people that are more technologically oriented, there is an abundance of online programs and even programs for your PDA that will aid in this task. See the resource section in this book for some suggested sites.

Case Study: Melissa

"I thought I was tracking my food intake."

Melissa was a twenty-eight-year-old woman who came to see me in September of 2006. She was married, owned a clothing store, and had an active two-year-old child. Her life was very busy and hectic. She weighed 202 pounds and was 61.5 inches tall, giving her a BMI score of 39. Melissa was clinically obese, tired, and had a poor self-image. She wanted to tackle weight loss and was ready to start.

Her lab test results and blood pressure were normal. There was no evidence of diabetes. I started Melissa on appetite suppressants and a 1400-calorie-per-day eating plan.

Melissa's follow-up was erratic. Sometimes, she would see me every two weeks. At other times, she wouldn't be in for two or three months. She was "trying," but her hectic life seemed to get in the way of her being able to reach a healthier weight.

By September of 2007, Melissa had lost thirteen pounds. I congratulated her on this loss, as it was an improvement that made a difference in her overall health. Melissa wasn't happy, though. For a month, she had been walking three miles a day, two to three times a week, and she wanted to see more progress for this hard work.

In a talk I had with Melissa, she admitted that she hadn't been keeping food records, but was "mentally" tracking her intake. She was skipping breakfast and snacking throughout the day. Further discussion revealed that, about three times a week, she would go out for beers after work with her colleagues. She had forgotten about this, and she wasn't tracking the beer calories. I explained to her that all calories count and that three pints of beer or more meant an extra 600+ calories, which was just about half of her calorie budget for an entire day. She was astounded!

Melissa gave this some thought and decided to make some changes. Two months later, she weighed in at 175 pounds, looked great, and, most importantly, felt much better. She had become diligent about keeping her food records and eating breakfast. She was now walking six mornings a week and had limited her social outings to two per week, when she would allow herself only one light beer. She also minimized the snacking that went along with the drinking.

Melissa had made a choice to change some of her habits. It wasn't painful. She was still able to socialize with her friends. Her improved energy level made it easier for her to keep up with her demanding schedule, and she felt much better about herself.

WHAT TO EAT, AND WHEN

I just don't know what to eat anymore!

—Patient

"Okay," you may say to yourself, "I know that I need to be calorie wise to bring about weight loss, but what should I eat?" Although all foods are fair game, you need nutritional balance in your day-to-day eating. The more nutritional balance you have in each meal, the more satisfied you will feel at the end of the meal. Include a protein source with each meal. Do you eat at least two fruits and three vegetables a day? Do not skip meals or go for long periods of time without eating. This behavior is not conducive to reaching and maintaining a healthy weight, as it often results in hunger and subsequent overeating, and even binging.

Spread your calorie intake throughout the day. Most people do well eating four to six small meals a day instead of two or three larger ones. By eating in this manner, your blood sugar will remain at a steadier level throughout the day. This prevents drops in glucose levels, which can result in fatigue, headaches, and irritability, as well as strong hunger and food cravings. Your metabolism functions more efficiently when you give your body food (fuel) throughout the day. The following is a suggested meal plan. Remember to stay within your calorie budget and drink plenty of water throughout the day.

BREAKFAST

Yogurt
Blueberries
Wheat toast with peanut butter
Orange juice
Coffee

MIDMORNING SNACK

Low-fat cheese
Granola bar

LUNCH

Turkey and cheese sandwich on wheat bread with lettuce, tomato, olives, and mustard
Pretzels
Apple
Lemonade

MIDAFTERNOON SNACK

Almonds
Grapes

DINNER

Grilled chicken
Asparagus
Salad
Rice pilaf
Iced tea

EVENING SNACK

Popcorn (non-buttered)

You can indeed choose to eat in the above manner. You also can exert control over your food choices by practicing "environmental" control. If you know that certain foods are just too difficult for you to resist, do not have them in your home, where you will hear them calling your name much too frequently. When a craving for candy hits and there is none around, you will think twice about having to go to the store to buy it. Clear your pantry, cabinets, and refrigerator shelves of unhealthy foods. Keep a variety of healthy foods available for snacking. One helpful aid is to keep these healthy snacks visible. Place them at the front of the refrigerator or pantry shelves. When you open the door, there they are, ready for the eating. These might include:

Low-fat string cheese	Frozen grapes
Cut-up fruits and vegetables Whole-grain crackers	Protein bars
Yogurt	Sugar-free Popsicles
Sugar-free puddings and gelatins	Hard-boiled eggs
Grape tomatoes	

It can be challenging when other members of your household freely enjoy the foods you find tempting. Talk with them and enlist their support. Ask them to keep these foods out of sight, and to eat them only when you're not around. If possible, ask them not to bring them home at all! Remember, it can be hard to get others to change, and your family members might even try to sabotage you. Keep the lines of communication open and try to discuss the situation honestly.

Let's talk about another way to exert environmental control. Many people are overwhelmed by their busy workweek and family responsibilities. You might be in such a hurry in the morning that you run out the door without breakfast and grab a cup of coffee on the way to work. You might buy lunch from a vending machine or restaurant and then rush back to your hectic pace at work. By the time the dinner hour rolls around, you're ravenous and have given no thought to what to eat for dinner. It becomes so easy to stop at a restaurant, bring home some fried chicken, or order a pizza.

This is another area in which you can make some beneficial changes. Spend some time on the weekend to plan your week and outline your breakfasts, lunches, and dinners. You can then go to the grocery store and purchase the ingredients for those meals. By doing this, you can easily prepare nutritious meals that are much more conducive to reaching and maintaining a healthy weight. You will most likely realize a cost savings, too.

So, to review, for health and weight loss:

1. **Aim for a variety of foods**. The fresher, the better. Minimize processed, convenience, and fast foods, which tend be higher in fat and sodium and contain many additives. Shop around the perimeter of the supermarket (where fresh foods are located) and evaluate the foods you are thinking of purchasing from the center aisles.

2. Based upon your appropriate caloric intake for the day, **plan for 50 percent of your calories to come from carbohydrates, 30 percent from fats, and the remaining 20 percent from protein.**

3. **Have carbohydrates, fats, and protein at each meal**. Doing this will keep your blood sugars steady and lead to greater satiety. This helps prevent hunger and overeating.

4. **Eat four to six times per day**. Including healthy midmorning and midafternoon snacks can help keep your blood sugars steady, increase energy, and minimize hunger.

5. **Choose more complex carbohydrates and fewer foods made from refined white flours**. Read food labels carefully. Avoid sugars such as high-fructose corn syrup. Eat lots of colorful fruits and vegetables that are raw, steamed, or roasted. Flavor foods with fresh herbs, lemon, lime, and low-fat salad dressings.

Carbohydrates have received a lot of attention over the past decade, and many people are concerned about "good" carbs, "bad" carbs, and the glycemic index. The glycemic index is a scale that measures the quantity of sugars in foods, with glucose topping the list. A food's "glycemic load" refers to its sugar content and to what other nutrients (such as fiber) it may contain that dilute the impact of the sugar. Why is this important?

Simple or refined carbohydrates are those starches that have a large amount of sugar in them. These include white flour products such as bread, enriched pasta and rice, waffles, bagels, sugared cereals, candy, pastries, and cookies. These simple carbohydrates are more easily and quickly digested, and—let's be honest—they can taste great. Ingesting these foods, however, results in a rapid spike in the blood glucose level. This subsequently results in more insulin being released by the pancreas. When this happens over and over, insulin resistance develops, which is a precursor to diabetes and obesity. In addition, prolonged elevated levels of insulin and glucose are ultimately toxic at the cellular level. This toxicity is the foundation for the development of diabetes type 2, coronary artery disease, degenerative disease processes, and certain cancers.

Complex carbohydrates like brown rice, bran products, oatmeal, barley, and other whole grains are converted to sugar more slowly, as they have more fiber in them. Adequate fiber in your diet can help you to feel fuller, thus controlling hunger. Diets high in fiber can moderate blood sugar levels, decrease cholesterol levels, and lead to a healthy GI tract.

6. **Choose fewer saturated fats and trans-hydrogenated fatty acids (margarines, butter, vegetable shortening, and lard) for your cardiovascular health.** These unhealthy fats can lead to heart and blood-vessel problems, and possibly to the development of certain cancers. Choose the healthier fatty acids found in extra-virgin olive oil, flaxseed oil, canola oil, nuts, salmon, sardines, and tuna. Look for a preponderance of omega-3s versus omega-6s. Omega-3s and omega-6s are essential fatty acids. This means that our bodies do not make these necessary acids—we need to get them from our diet or supplements. They serve as building blocks for hormones and chemicals that control our immune system, blood clotting, and cellular growth. Remember, not all fats are bad, and we need them to survive.

Omega-3 fatty acids are found in fish such as salmon, sardines, mackerel, and bluefish. Omega-6 fatty acids are much more abundant in our diet. They are found in seeds and nuts, and the oils from these foods. Soybean, corn, safflower, and cottonseed oils provide omega-6 fatty acids.

Both fatty acids are important in helping us to have healthy skin and hair, lower cholesterol, and proper immune function. But too much of the omega-6s can result in increased inflammation, which can lead to heart disease, certain forms of cancer, and autoimmune diseases. Therefore, cut back on fast foods and processed foods, which are high in omega-6. Boost your intake of omega-3s by eating more fish, nuts, and flaxseed. A higher intake of omega-3s can result in decreased blood pressure, decreased cholesterol, and, I believe, a decreased risk of heart disease and cancer.

Remember, our bodies *do* need fats to survive and function.

7. **Eat adequate protein throughout the day.** Most protein in our diets comes from meat, poultry, and seafood. Other good protein sources are beans, soy products, yogurt, cottage cheese, and nuts. A quick way to estimate your protein needs during weight loss is to take your weight and multiply by 0.4. This formula will give you a general idea of your daily protein needs in grams per day. For example, a man weighing 200 pounds would need about 80 grams of protein per day. A woman weighing 160 pounds would need about

64 grams. A 300-pound person needs about 120 grams of protein per day. Of course, this assumes that you have healthy liver and kidney function. If you have any health concerns or medical conditions, it is always wise to discuss dietary changes with your doctor.

8.   **Strive to eat about forty grams of fiber per day.** This can come from fresh fruits, vegetables, berries, and whole-grain cereals and breads.

9.   **Drink plenty of water and noncaffeinated beverages**. Hydrate your tissues! Caffeinated beverages and alcohol pull water out of your cells and actually result in dehydration. Thus, these should be limited.

10.   If you wish (and I do recommend it), **take a vitamin/mineral supplement** that includes vitamin C, vitamin E, selenium, vitamin D, CoQ-10, and alpha-lipoic acid. Also consider taking a low-dose aspirin each day for cardiac health. Because so many people eat processed and convenience foods, I suggest supplementation in order to ensure that you are getting essential nutrients. CoQ-10 enzyme and alpha-lipoic acid are antioxidants that are important in cell-to-cell communication. Supplementation with these antioxidants and fish-oil capsules can help boost your immune system and decrease the risk of heart disease and cancer. Of course, though, any supplementation you might be considering should first be discussed with your doctor.

GOALS

Let's spend a minute talking about your weight goals. If you need and want to lose fifty pounds, and this is realistic, develop a plan. It can be discouraging to focus only on the fifty pounds. The number can seem so formidable. Break it down into attainable short-term targets. Start with the goal of losing ten pounds over a specific time period. Remember, make your goal *realistic*. If it isn't, you're more likely to become discouraged when you deviate from your plan, or if your weight goes up a pound or two. You will be more likely to give up.

Plan a ten-pound weight loss over ten or fifteen weeks. This is all that you need to lose—not fifty pounds, only ten. When you reach this goal, you can begin to strive for the *next* ten pounds in a similar manner. Over time, you will reach your overall goal of fifty pounds of weight loss.

If you don't reach your target of ten pounds in a realistic time period, be patient with yourself. Don't give up. Reevaluate your food intake and activity level. Where might you be able to make some changes? If you were able to lose five pounds instead of ten, congratulate yourself. Your loss may be progressing a little more slowly than you'd like, but your weight *is* going in the right direction. It might take you a year to lose ten pounds, and that's okay. It's still better than *gaining* ten pounds. Most likely, you will have developed some healthy habits that will enable you to maintain that ten-pound loss and be able to go forth to lose more. Remember, this is not a race. This is about becoming healthier for life.

Now, let's discuss the other factor in the weight-loss equation—*exercise*.

EXERCISE

> *Obstacles are those frightful things you see when you take your eyes off your goal.*
>
> —Henry Ford

The thought of exercise can be intimidating to overweight people. "It hurts to exercise." "I'm embarrassed by my body and don't want others to see me." The self-sabotaging thoughts can go on and on. See if you can relate to some of the following excuses people make for not exercising.

It's too hot outside	I have to take my children to events
It's too cold outside	I have company
I'm too busy	I went on vacation
I'm bored	I have a cold
It's raining outside	My exercise partner is sick
It's too sunny	I don't like to exercise
The sun's not out	Exercise is boring
I'm tired	People will look at me and talk about me
I don't have a dog to walk	I want to lose weight first
I have no room for exercise equipment	I'm too awkward to move around in public

Everyone can always find a reason for not exercising. However, let's reframe the discussion and begin to think of *moving the body*. The body is a machine and is meant to be used. It is very difficult to lose weight and keep it off through dietary restriction alone. It is essential to increase your activity level, especially during weight loss, to keep lean muscle mass. In addition, consistent activity leads to increased muscle mass.

Muscle is more metabolically active than fat tissue and therefore will result in an increased metabolic rate over the long term. For example, one pound of muscle mass burns approximately thirty calories per day. On the other hand, one pound of fat burns only about *three* calories per day. More muscle mass is desirable, as it will help you to maintain your new weight.

Activity has many benefits beyond weight loss. These include a greater sense of well-being due to the balancing and regulation of hormones and body chemicals, stress reduction, increased metabolic rate, increased body tone, and improved sleep. When you exercise in conjunction with eating in a healthier manner, you will have a greater chance of success in losing weight and in maintaining your new weight.

It is important to find activities that you enjoy. It doesn't make sense to vow to walk on a treadmill three times a week for thirty minutes if you hate the treadmill. This is not something you will be able to maintain. It's far better to look for ways to increase activity in your day-to-day life. Find enjoyable activities that will allow you to be more active.

I suggest wearing a pedometer. A pedometer keeps track of the steps you walk each day and is a pretty good objective measurement of your degree of physical activity. Clip your pedometer to your belt or waistband, right in front of your hip. Put it on in the morning after getting dressed and wear it all day. It will take into account the steps walked at home, at work, when you are out and about, and when you are exercising. At the end of the day, record the number of steps you've taken. It's easy to put this number into your Food/Exercise Record, and it will help you calculate results. You'll quickly be able to see how parking the car a little farther away from your destination, taking the stairs instead of the elevator, and walking to the mailbox instead of driving increase the number of steps taken.

Two thousand steps are roughly equal to one mile. The ultimate goal for weight loss is to reach 10,000 steps per day. However, if you find that your daily activity gives you only about 4000 steps per day, increase the number of steps you take in increments of 500 until you reach the 10,000 mark. Most people will need to incorporate some form of structured activity into their days to reach 10,000 steps.

Table 6—Sample Exercise Record

Exercise Record	Activity	Pedometer Steps
Monday	½-mile walk before breakfast	1000
	Up and down from desk during the day	3000
	Rode bicycle in evening for 20 minutes	3000
		TOTAL = 7000

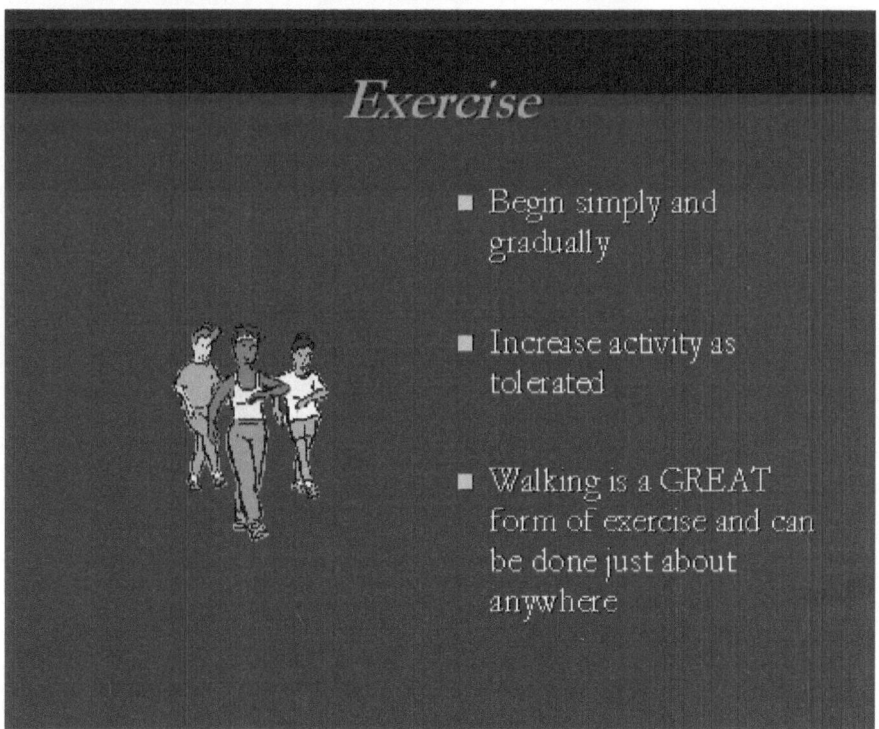

Figure 6
Benefits of Walking as Exercise

A word of caution—your pedometer readings may be falsely elevated by a bumpy car ride, when worn while horseback riding, or when driving a piece of heavy equipment. Keep checking your pedometer for accuracy and make the necessary adjustments. Pedometers will not register steps taken when cycling or swimming. Your pedometer readings could even be incorrect due to the type of clothing you wear. Waistbands that roll, and heavier, thicker material such as denim may make it difficult for the pedometer to track your steps, as it is not in close contact with the body. Again, keep checking for accuracy and make the necessary adjustments.

For those of you who have great difficulty with exercise because of your size or overall health condition, think of other ways in which you might be able to increase your movement. If you're in a wheelchair, are you able to move your arms and stretch daily? If you're on oxygen, are you able to walk across the room? Little steps and a little movement count, and are the starting points of your weight-loss journey.

Certainly, structured activity is beneficial and should be a goal for anyone trying to improve health. We live in such a sedentary society that we need to make an effort to incorporate exercise into our day-to-day lives. Research has shown that 92 percent of people who are able to maintain a healthy weight exercise regularly. On the other hand, only 34 percent of those who regain weight exercise regularly.

Walking is a wonderful form of activity. Begin slowly. If you can only walk for five minutes at a time, so be it. As you lose weight and improve your aerobic conditioning, you will be able to step up the pace and increase the distance walked. Add a minute or two to your walk every week. Before you know it, you'll be walking thirty minutes a day and enjoying it!

In addition to participating in an activity that improves your cardiovascular health, choose other exercises that will increase your muscle mass, such as resistance training or weightlifting. As you develop more muscle mass, you will increase your metabolic rate for the long term. Remember, muscle is a much more metabolically active tissue than fat. Thus, the ideal combination of activity is one blending some form of aerobic activity (walking, biking, swimming, dancing) with light weightlifting, use of resistance bands, Pilates, or yoga. This combination will offer you the optimal opportunity to shed pounds and maintain a healthy weight.

Think about your feelings towards increased activity. If they are negative, try to frame them in a more positive light. Remember, exercise doesn't mean putting on spandex and going to the gym. It means increased movement for overall improved health. Reframe those negative excuses as positive statements:

Since it's cold outside, I'll wear my hat and gloves when I go for my walk.

My exercise partner is sick, but I can still go to the mall and do my thirty minutes of walking by myself.

I don't have room in the house for exercise equipment, but I can get down on the floor and stretch. I have a radio and can put on some music and move to it.

I can set my alarm for fifteen minutes earlier each morning, get up, and walk on the treadmill for fifteen minutes.

Instead of using the elevator, I'll walk the two flights of stairs to my office each day.

Make a commitment to yourself to be physically active for thirty minutes each day. This can include mowing the lawn with a push mower instead of a riding mower, walking the golf course instead of riding in a cart, parking the car a little farther away from your destination, getting up from your desk and delivering your message to a co-worker in person instead of sending him an e-mail, or walking to a nearby restaurant for lunch instead of driving.

Just as you have a goal of losing a certain number of pounds, you should establish some activity goals as well. It's very effective to keep a journal and write things down accurately. Every weekend, take a few minutes to review the upcoming week's schedule. Write down on your calendar specific dates and times when you will exercise. This will solidify your commitment—it becomes an appointment that you must keep, just like any other. You are more likely to accomplish something when it is written down on your to-do list.

Remember, small steps add up. Little changes along the way do make a big difference. If you truly want to reach and maintain a healthier weight, increased activity is not just an option—it is a *necessity*.

Research is showing that even 5 to 10 percent weight loss can result in a significant improvement in health and a reduction in risk factors (Knowler et al. 2002, 393–403). For example, if you are a forty-year-old man who is seventy-two inches tall and weighs 275 pounds, losing *and keeping off* between fourteen and twenty-five pounds will greatly improve your overall health and lower your health risks. Would it be ideal for you to lose more weight than this? Yes, and that probably is possible. However, if not, and if you can stay at your new weight—even though you are not at your "ideal" weight as listed on a piece of paper—you have still achieved a great success and improved your health. This is the goal to strive for. *You can do it!*

DOCTOR-PRESCRIBED MEDICATION

Many of my patients elect to use prescription weight-loss medications. Medication can play an important role in the treatment of your overweight condition. Remember, we are trying to tweak those metabolic and biochemical factors that are otherwise beyond your control. There are several medications that help with weight loss.

Sibutramine (which goes by the brand name Meridia) is an appetite suppressant that affects the brain chemicals norepinephrine and serotonin. These chemicals affect hunger and satiety (feeling full and satisfied) so that one experiences decreased hunger and cravings for foods. Meridia also can slightly enhance one's metabolism. A common side effect from Meridia can be an elevation in blood pressure, so if you take Meridia, you should be seeing your physician and having your blood pressure monitored regularly.

Phentermine (Adipex, Fastin) and diethylproprion (Tenuate) are two other appetite suppressants that primarily affect norepinephrine and dopamine, respectively. They result in decreased hunger, decreased cravings for foods, and feeling full more quickly. Their primary side effects can include restlessness, dry mouth, elevated blood pressure, and sleeplessness.

Orlistat (Xenical) prevents the body from absorbing about one-third of the fat content of any one meal. This fat remains undigested, so the body is ultimately taking in fewer calories. Side effects can include diarrhea and excess gas.

Alli is an FDA-approved over-the-counter version of Xenical. It prevents the body from absorbing about a quarter of the fat you eat. Undigested fat cannot be reabsorbed and thus passes through the intestines. Again, side effects can include excessive gas, oily spotting, and diarrhea.

I do not recommend the use of any of the multitude of over-the-counter diet pills. They come with a lot of big promises, but they can have detrimental effects on your body. Many contain stimulants that can increase your heart rate and blood pressure. Furthermore, they usually don't work, cost a lot of money, and certainly don't help with long-term weight maintenance.

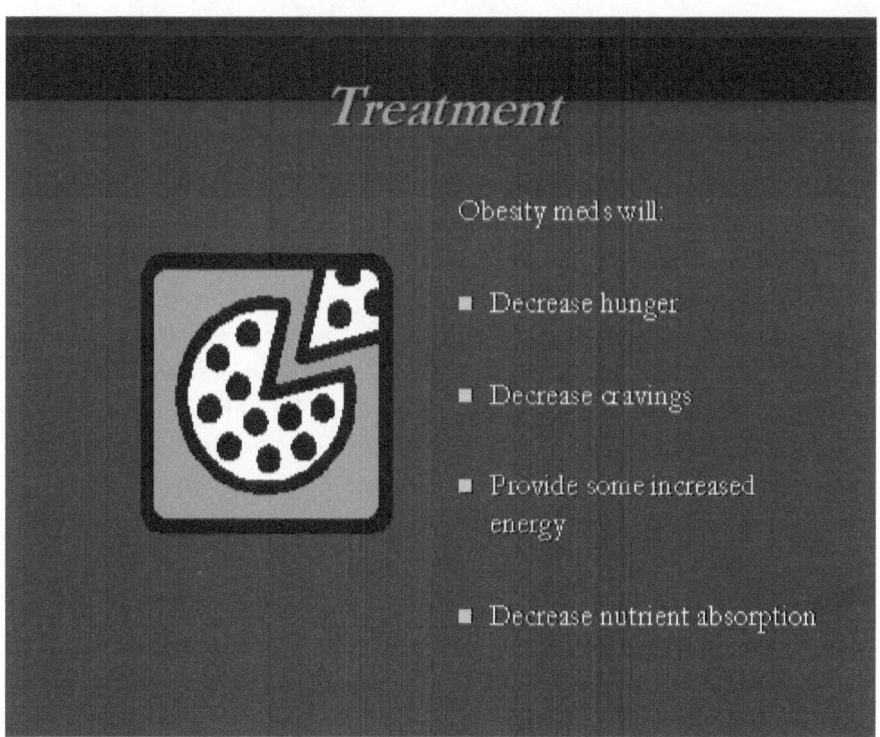

Figure 7
Benefits of Obesity Medications

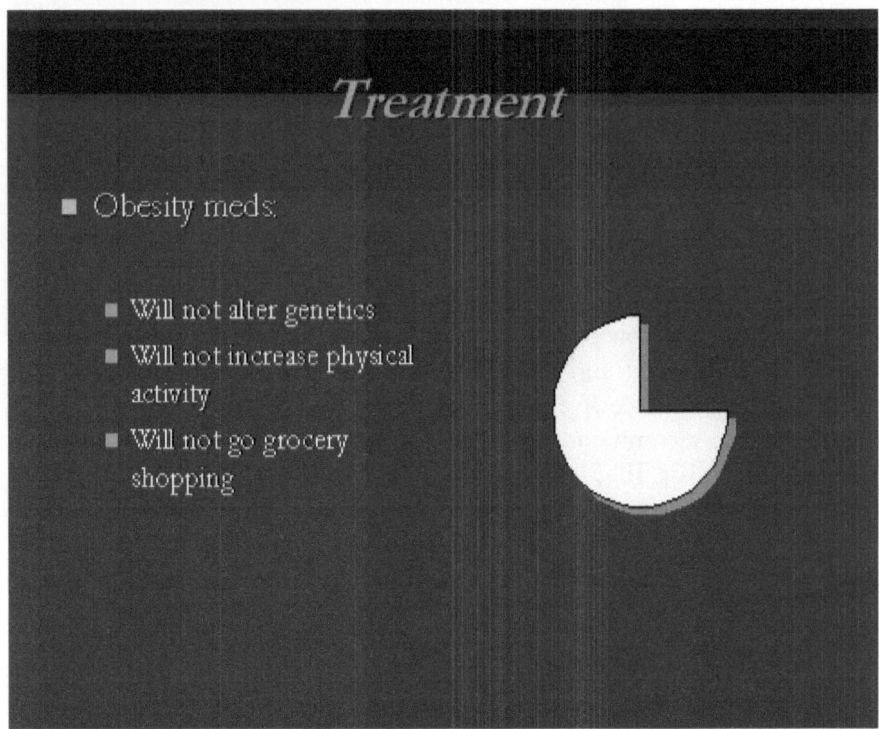

Figure 8
Limitations of Obesity Medications

There are many other prescription medications in the research pipeline, in various stages of development. The more we learn about the biology and biochemistry of weight regulation, the greater the possibility for the development of medications that target specific areas for treatment. Which medication you use (if any) will depend upon your medical and weight history. If you again look at the biology of weight regulation, you can realize that your use of medication might be long-term. We are looking at weight regulation as a physiological process, in which medication can indeed play a role. Remember, though, that weight-loss medications are *not* miracle drugs or cures—they are helpful *tools*. Medications should be used under the supervision of your health-care provider, and only in the appropriate doses. Do not rely on medications alone to help you lose weight. You need to do your part as well, by committing to lifestyle change.

Case Study: Lucy

"I don't feel as if I'm on a diet."

Lucy is a forty-five-year-old woman who has struggled with her weight for most of her life. She weighed 170 pounds when she graduated from high school and 210 pounds by the age of thirty (after having had two children). Any diet she tried would result in some weight loss, but she found that she couldn't sustain the rigid eating plans required. She would "blow my diet, call it quits," and regain her lost weight, and then some.

Lucy did not have a history of anorexia, bulimia, or binge-eating disorder. However, her eating habits were poor, and she craved carbohydrates. Evenings seemed to be most problematic for her. After a full dinner, she would find herself eating an extra piece of pie, then perhaps looking for some chips, and finally having a dish of ice cream before bed.

At forty-five, Lucy now weighed 250 pounds. She was sixty-six inches tall, giving her a BMI of forty-two. Her cholesterol was creeping up, and her lab results showed early indications of diabetes. She was also taking a blood-pressure medication. Lucy was motivated to lose weight for health reasons. She also wanted to feel more energetic and be able to keep up with her children.

My evaluation showed that Lucy's body was 44 percent fat, and that her RMR was 1810. Given Lucy's history of carbohydrate cravings, I started her on phentermine and Tenuate, with careful monitoring of her blood pressure in conjunction with an eating plan of 1400 calories per day and a graduated walking program.

Again, I stressed that this was not a diet, but the beginning of a lifestyle change. All food was fair game, but, of course, the goal was for her to have overall improved nutrition. Within three months, Lucy had lost twenty-two pounds and was walking four days a week for thirty minutes at a time. Her lab results had normalized. She reported that her cravings were gone. She continued to work on healthy food choices and had a protein source at each meal. According to Lucy, "This makes sense. I'm learning that there isn't really a 'bad' food. If I want a piece of chocolate, I indulge, but I'm able to control my portion and stay within my calorie balance. I don't feel as if I'm dieting. This is the way I plan to eat forever!"

After one year, Lucy had lost sixty-eight pounds, her BMI was 31.5, and she had discontinued her blood-pressure medication. Her walking had increased to one hour per day, five days a week, and she had even begun to do some running. Eighteen months after starting her weight-loss journey, Lucy had completed five 5k and 10k races, in which she did a combination of walking and running. Lucy told me that she had reframed her thinking. "I don't think of myself as a fat, middle-aged mother anymore. I now think of myself as an athlete!"

BARIATRIC SURGERY

No discussion of treatment would be complete without mentioning bariatric surgery. Bariatric surgery provides a viable option for people struggling with morbid obesity (as defined by having a BMI greater than forty) and who have been unable to attain and maintain a healthier weight. The surgery is a major procedure, and not one to be entered into lightly. Each individual must determine whether the benefits exceed the risks.

Currently, the gold standard for weight-loss surgery is the Roux-En-Y procedure, or gastric bypass surgery (GBS). This surgery can be done via the open method, or, more commonly, the laparoscopic method. GBS involves decreasing the size of the stomach and repositioning a part of the small intestine. The result is that one will take in less food because the capacity

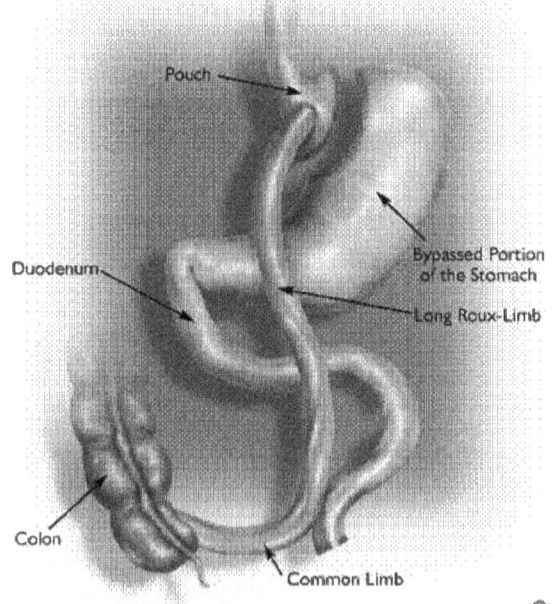

Figure 9 Gastric Bypass Roux-en-Y
Ethicon Endo-Surgery, Inc. grants limited license for use of the Roux-en-Y image as provided by Riley King for use as requested. Please attribute to image "Courtesy of Ethicon Endo-Surgery Inc."

of the stomach is smaller. This is known as the *restrictive* component of the surgery. There will also be decreased calorie absorption because of the rerouting of the small intestine. This is called the *malabsorptive* component.

Bariatric surgery is not for everyone wanting to lose weight. It does not constitute a quick and easy fix. It is for those people with a BMI of forty or greater and who are 100 pounds or more overweight. Many people with this degree of obesity also have other chronic medical conditions, including diabetes type 2, heart disease, high blood pressure, sleep apnea, arthritis, and high cholesterol. These conditions are typically greatly improved, and are often even entirely resolved, after the surgery and subsequent weight loss.

GBS is an excellent tool to help you manage your weight. However, to optimize this tool, you still need to work at healthy weight management and increased activity *over the long term*. Because the surgical method is more drastic than medical weight loss, it is imperative not to choose it lightly. Research the topic, find a qualified bariatric surgery team, and commit to adequate preoperative preparation and postoperative follow-up. Investing the time in preparing for the surgery and committing to postoperative follow-up will give you the greatest chance for successful weight loss and the maintenance of your new weight.

The following resources may be helpful to you in researching bariatric surgery:

www.asbs.org

www.obesitysurgery.com

www.obesityhelp.com

www.bariatricedge.com

www.BariatricSupportCenter.com

www.lapband.com

Is bariatric surgery effective? Success depends on many variables, including age, weight before surgery, activity level, commitment to following postoperative dietary and exercise guidelines, and participating in regular follow-up care. Motivation to maintain your healthy weight and support from family, friends, and co-workers is also important. Realize that bariatric surgery does *not* fix the emotional aspects of eating. Thus, ongoing support and appropriate long-term follow-up become even more important.

After surgery, most patients lose weight rapidly. By the end of the first postoperative year, the rate of weight loss slows but does typically continue for another six to twelve months. By the two-year mark, people who have had the surgery have lost the amount of weight that their body wishes to lose. Some studies have shown that patients will lose about 30 to 50 percent of their excess weight after six months and 77 percent of their excess weight by the twelve-month mark. Other studies have shown that most patients can keep off about 50 to 60 percent of their lost weight over an extended period of time. The national average for a bariatric surgical patient is a loss of about 65 percent of excess body weight. Only about 5 percent of people who have gastric bypass surgery will reach a "normal" weight. Because of the complexity of weight regulation, the body tends to reach a new set point and stay there. Again, this stabilization point is most likely not the "ideal" number found on a height/weight chart. However, the weight loss will undoubtedly result in a marked improvement in health.

Bariatric surgery is not a magic bullet. It is a major surgical procedure that typically does not result in one reaching an "ideal" body weight. In time, some of the lost weight might even be regained. However, it is still the best tool we currently have to bring about a significant amount of weight loss in the morbidly obese, and the one that offers the greatest possibility for them to keep it off. Bariatric surgery is not an "easy way out." It is a life-saving and life-changing procedure that results in the improvement or resolution of many obesity-related medical complications. Despite the risks involved, I haven't had a single patient who has regretted having had the surgery. Many people even celebrate the anniversary of their surgery as a commemoration of the beginning of their new life.

Gastric banding is another bariatric surgical option. This involves an adjustable silicone ring that is surgically placed around the upper part of the stomach. The inner part of the ring is filled with saline. When this ring is inflated, a smaller stomach pouch results. The band also controls the stoma (opening) linking the upper and lower parts of the stomach. This reduces the capacity of the stomach and causes food to move more slowly between its two sections. Thus, you take in less food and feel full more readily.

The procedure is typically done via a laparoscope. After the lap band is placed and secured, tubing is used to connect it to a port that has been fixed beneath the skin of the abdomen. The surgeon then inflates or deflates the ring by injecting or draining saline through the port. These post surgical adjustments are done periodically, depending upon the degree of weight loss and symptoms a patient may be experiencing.

Again, the lap band is not a quick fix. Patients who elect to undergo this procedure require appropriate follow-up care. Nutrition and exercise remain important parts of the equation for healthy weight loss and maintenance.

QUESTIONS TO ASK YOURSELF

1. What are my weight-loss goals?

2. Do I eat breakfast?

3. How many grams of protein do I take in each day?

4. How will I incorporate my favorite foods into my healthy eating plan?

5. How many calories should I take in each day?

6. How am I increasing my activity?

7. How many days a week can I commit to keeping food and exercise records?

8. What are three ways that I can increase my physical activity?

9. Who will be my support people along my weight-loss journey?

MOVING FORWARD

1. Keep food and exercise records.

2. Portion control is important.

3. Calories do count.

4. Eat breakfast.

5. Have a protein source at each meal.

6. All foods are fair game—but in moderation.

7. Weight-loss medication, if used appropriately, is a helpful tool.

8. Aim for a slow and steady weight loss over time.

9. Increased activity is a necessity.

10. Wear a pedometer.

11. Strive for a fit and healthy body.

5

Why Do I Weigh What I Do?

○ ○
Why am I so overweight? I really don't eat that much.

—Patient

We all know people who seem to be able to eat anything they want and never gain a pound. Conversely, we know of others who seem to gain an extra five pounds by just *looking* at food. Likewise, there are those people who can exercise three days a week for twenty minutes at a time and maintain a healthy weight, while others have to sweat it out for an hour a day, seven days a week, to barely "hold on." Why is this so?

Medical research is helping us to realize the enormous complexity involved in weight regulation. Certainly, what you eat and what you do for activity are important. However, there are genetic, biochemical, metabolic, hormonal, cultural, environmental, and psychological factors involved as well. Some of these things are in your control, *but others are not*. Let's take a look at some of these factors.

GENETICS, BIOCHEMISTRY, AND HORMONES

At this time, over four hundred genes have been identified that are involved in weight regulation. These genes are expressed to varying degrees from person to person. Even a slight change in one of these genes can result in significant obesity. They are involved in the production, release, and regulation of various chemicals and hormones in the body. These chemicals and hormones, in turn, communicate with each other in various parts of the body to ultimately determine the body's weight.

For example, the *Ob* gene helps to direct the production of a hormone called *leptin*, which occurs in the fat cell. When leptin is released, it travels via the bloodstream to certain areas of the brain and helps us determine how full we feel after eating. It also acts as a barometer of sorts, telling the brain how much fat mass is stored in the body.

Another chemical of importance in weight regulation is *ghrelin*. Ghrelin is a hormone that is manufactured in cells in the GI tract. It sends messages to the brain that tell the brain that we are hungry. The brain, in turn, activates other chemical messengers that trigger feelings of hunger and desire for food. It is interesting to note that after people have had gastric bypass surgery, their ghrelin levels decrease. They do not tend to experience much hunger for the next twelve to eighteen months. However, after that time, their ghrelin levels rise, and they begin to feel hungry again. We do not know why this happens.

Leptin and ghrelin are affected by other factors as well. Several studies have shown a relationship between weight regulation and the duration of sleep. A study conducted at the University of Chicago revealed that subjects receiving four hours of sleep compared to those receiving more than four hours of sleep per night exhibited a change in leptin and ghrelin levels. During sleep restriction, there was an 18 percent decrease in leptin and a 28 percent increase in ghrelin levels. Likewise, there was a 24 percent increase in hunger, especially for higher-calorie foods like cookies, cakes, candy, and chips (Spiegel 2004, 885–886).

Additional research is being done in women to investigate the effects of estrogen and its relationship to weight and fat deposition. Many women will experience weight gain and more fat accumulation around the waist after menopause. Why is this so? It appears that there are estrogen receptors in the brain—specifically, in the hypothalamus—that are important in the control of food intake and energy expenditure. In animal studies, when these receptors are destroyed or blocked, the animals begin to eat much more food and gain weight at an accelerated rate. Thus, given the declining level of estrogen that occurs at menopause, those receptors in the hypothalamus may not be adequately activated. Hence, this may be a possible explanation for the associated weight gain and fat accumulation.

Again, there is no one simple cause of obesity. There are multiple systems involved. What we *do* know is that even a very slight change along any of these multiple pathways can result in increasing weight, and even severe obesity. The genetic variations from person to person help explain why some people cannot reach their "ideal" body weight. Thus, one cannot necessarily will oneself to be a size six when one's genetics are dictating a body size of fourteen, nor can one will oneself to have a belt size of thirty-two when one's genetics have dictated a size thirty-six. As one's genes determine eye color, hair color, and shape of one's nose, *one's genes are the foundation for determining body weight and shape.* Your genes also determine your metabolic rate. Let's spend some time talking about metabolism.

METABOLISM

Metabolism—many people who are overweight doubt that they even have one! Well, we *all* do. Some people's engines just burn a little hotter than others. Metabolism refers to the body's way of combining the nutrients we digest with oxygen to produce the energy required to keep our bodies functioning. This energy is measured in terms of calories. The resting metabolic rate (RMR) is the minimum number of calories that the body requires to function. In other words, if you woke up in the morning, remained in bed, and didn't do much else, your body would still require energy to keep your heart beating, your lungs breathing, and your brain functioning. This is the RMR. The RMR accounts for about 75 percent of a person's daily calorie needs. The remaining 25 percent is determined by one's overall activity level.

Each person's metabolism is as unique as his blood pressure. It is the metabolic rate that explains why one person can "look at food and gain five pounds" and another can eat "whatever he wants and not gain weight." Just as your blood pressure and cholesterol can be measured, so can the RMR. This can be done with an instrument (called a calorimeter) designed for this purpose. If possible, find a health-care provider, clinic, hospital, or even an athletic club that can perform this measurement. The information will be quite valuable to you. When you know your RMR, you can determine the calorie intake level that will lead to weight loss. There are standardized formulas to help you determine this number. However, they do not take into account the genetic differences between individuals. For more information about determining your resting metabolic rate, refer to chapter 4 of this book.

Our unique metabolisms do indeed present us with a challenge. Metabolically, as one strives to lose weight, the body's primal mechanisms want to push that person back up to his original weight, which is called the "set point." You may have come across this term before. A long time ago, when our ancestors lived on the savannah and were hunters and gatherers, their bodies used this protective mechanism to keep them alive. When there was an abundance of food, people would eat as much as they could and store the extra calories (energy) as fat. During times of famine, the body's metabolism would slow down to preserve critical functioning (heartbeat, brain function, breathing, and so on) and use the stored energy to survive. This was a fairly tightly regulated and efficient mechanism, and essential for survival.

However, in our society today, starvation is typically not a threat, and most of us aren't too physically active. Our bodies don't know these things, though. When a person begins to lower his calorie intake, there is usually an initial weight loss. Then, the rate of loss slows and eventually comes to a halt. The body has interpreted the change in diet as a sign of starvation and has slowed down the metabolism. This makes it difficult to get to that "ideal" body weight. All is not lost, though. You can counter this mechanism with healthy eating patterns, consistent activity, and *gradual* weight loss. Remember also that muscle is a more metabolically active tissue than fat.

This has by no means been an exhaustive review of the biochemistry of weight regulation, but has merely been meant to give you an idea of the complex interactions between the fat cell, the GI tract, and the brain. Science is still in the early stages of understanding these issues and has much to learn.

Oh! you might be thinking, *So being overweight isn't my fault. It's all in my genes!* Not quite. While you cannot change your genes, you *can* exert control over your environment. Remember, as is often pointed out, genetics may load the gun, but the environment pulls the trigger.

ENVIRONMENT AND CULTURE

One's environment and culture are important to think about—home, workplace, school, family, friends, and peers. We can control how we live in and respond to our environment. It is in this area that you can begin to modify your lifestyle and, in time, develop some healthier habits that will lead you to a healthier weight.

Begin by thinking about your personal family history. This is where you first developed your thoughts, attitudes, and behavior regarding food, eating, and activity. Our ethnic and socioeconomic background dictated what food was brought into the home, how it was prepared, and how much of it we ate. Many of us grew up in "meat and potatoes" families or in families whose foods were fried in butter or lard. Others grew up in vegetarian families or in cultures that emphasized vegetables alongside small amounts of protein. Many of us belong to the "clean your plate" club.

Were desserts a part of your everyday pattern or reserved for special occasions? What significance was placed upon these foods? Did your family ski, hike, or swim for fun or did your family watch movies and TV for fun and relaxation? Was there and emphasis on "dieting" or were you told as a child that you were "getting heavy and needed to lose weight?" As you think about questions like this, you will begin to recognize why you make some of the food and activity choices you make today. With this increased awareness, you can begin to make changes. You will no longer need to eat or prepare something because "that's the way we've always done it."

Today, in our society, we have an abundance of food that is high in calories, low in cost, and easy to obtain. These foods aren't always healthy for us, yet they are almost always present for the purchasing. As we have discussed, many of us skip breakfast, make a mad dash out the door, and stop for a latte or mocha on our way to work. The office vending machine is often the provider of the midmorning snack, and even lunch for some. Others work all morning and afternoon at their desks never stopping for lunch. When dinnertime comes around, many people haven't even given a second thought to what they will have. It then becomes easier to stop at a fast-food restaurant, order a pizza, or just eat a bowl of cereal.

When we couple these habits with living a sedentary life, they can result in a weight-gain nightmare. We will now talk about how to think about these issues and respond differently to them. It's all about making choices. It is not as hard as you think, and I will guide you. Making even small changes to daily life can result in a healthier and sustainable weight.

It is important to remember that dealing with a weight problem is a chronic situation. Once you have a weight issue, you will *always* have a weight issue. It is very similar to having diabetes. Once you develop diabetes, you will always have a propensity for diabetes. You cannot ignore the need for a healthy lifestyle, the use of appropriate medication, and self-care. Being overweight is no different. The battle to reach and maintain a healthy weight does not end. There is no quick fix or easy answer. Weight loss and maintenance requires persistence and diligence, but it doesn't have to be painful or about denial. *Obesity cannot be cured, but it can be controlled, and you* can *reach your goal of a healthier weight.*

Many overweight and obese people are thought of as being "weak-willed" and "lazy." This is absolutely untrue! Being overweight or obese is not due to poor character or lack of willpower. Overweight people are not "bad" people. People struggling with their weight have complex metabolic and medical issues. It's time that society addresses the problem in this way. I encourage you to seek medical help with your weight, just as you would for high blood pressure, menstrual cramps, a torn knee ligament, depression, or cancer. Let's work through this step by step.

And, incidentally, I'm not sure that I've ever known anyone who can *really* eat whatever and whenever he or she wants and never gain any weight!

Case Study: Molly

"Everybody in my family is heavy."

Molly was a thirty-two-year-old woman seeking help with weight loss. She told me that she had always struggled with her weight and was overweight even as a child. "I was always the fat kid in class." Molly recalls weighing 210 pounds when she graduated from high school, and then 250 pounds when she graduated from college. Molly was 5'4" in height and her BMI was 43.

She tried to exercise and had been on many diets. She was a lifelong member of Weight Watchers. Any weight she had ever lost, she regained, and then some. Molly said that she was at her wits' end. She now weighed 300 pounds and was miserable. "I have friends who can eat anything they want and never gain an ounce. They don't even go to the gym. I look at food and gain ten pounds!"

In a conversation I had with Molly, she revealed that "everybody in my family is heavy." She had two aunts who had had bariatric surgery. Her mother weighed 400 pounds, and her little sister, who was twenty-five, now weighed 230 pounds. Molly's father had died of a heart attack when he was fifty-five years old. He had weighed 375 pounds and had had diabetes that was difficult to control. Molly pulled a picture out of her wallet and showed it to me. It was picture of her with her sister, mother, aunt, and grandmother. It was uncanny how alike they all looked—not only in their facial features, but in their body shape and size as well.

Molly also told me that food had always been a big part of their family life. Her mother was a great cook, and each meal was a feast. In fact, in her family, if you didn't clean your plate and have seconds, you offended the cook.

Molly had numerous challenges facing her. Her obesity had such a strong genetic component that we had to talk about setting realistic goals. Molly would never be a size six, but she could reach a healthier weight and stay there.

QUESTIONS TO ASK YOURSELF

1. Who in my family is overweight or obese?

2. Do I struggle with constantly thinking about and craving food?

3. What do I like about my body?

4. What don't I like about my body?

5. What are my eating patterns?

6. What are my activity patterns?

7. How do I spend my time after dinner every evening?

MOVING FORWARD

1. There are many factors involved in weight regulation.

2. Genetic, metabolic, biochemical, and hormonal factors are beyond your control.

3. Obesity is not due to a lack of willpower or poor character.

4. What you choose to eat and do for activity is in your control.

6

Restaurants, Parties, Holidays, and Family Gatherings—Help!

Your stomach shouldn't be a waist basket.

—Author unknown

Occasions like parties, holidays, and family gatherings are a part of everyday life and a great source of pleasure and fun (most of the time). At the same time, they can inspire fear and dread in a person trying to achieve a healthier weight, because we don't often pay attention to what we are eating, or how much. We are also often subject to the pressures of our family and friends to "try this" or "have a little more." Many people will avoid these experiences altogether, for fear of "falling off of the diet."

Remember, though, you *are not dieting*. You are getting healthier. It is inevitable that there will be holiday parties, family celebrations, business travel, and restaurant eating in your life. None of these occasions, however, needs to be an excuse for an eating frenzy. Let's talk about how to deal with this, because you are a social person, you enjoy the conversation, and you want to be able to participate in life, even though you are on a weight-loss journey. These two aspects of your life are not mutually exclusive. You can learn to manage your weight in the midst of enjoying life!

TIPS FOR DINING OUT

Here are a few tips to use when dining out. When you go to a restaurant, look at the menu. Which foods are broiled, baked, or grilled? Which entrees are served with heavy cream sauces? Which are not? What side dishes are available? What beverages are offered? What are the desserts? (Yes, you *can* have dessert!) Be wise about your choices. Instead of the sixteen-ounce prime rib, opt for the salmon or halibut. If you really want that prime rib, how about choosing the eight-ounce portion with a salad and omitting the potato with sour cream? If you have your eye on a certain dessert, you may want to choose a lighter-calorie entree to save some calories for the end of the meal.

Opt for only one piece of bread, without the butter. If you think that the bread and butter might be too tempting, ask your server not to bring bread to the table at all. Salads with dressings on the side are great appetizers. This way, you can take a forkful of your salad and dip it into the dressing. Choose the steamed or grilled vegetables instead of the potato or rice, as the former tend to have fewer calories.

If you don't see healthier options on the menu, ask whether they can be made to order. Many restaurants are willing and able to accommodate your needs and often will be able to serve you grilled fish with lemon wedges on the side, without the cream sauce advertised on the menu. Another helpful hint is to eat only half of your meal and take the rest home to enjoy for lunch the next day. Many establishments serve overlarge portions of food—much more than we truly need. When your plate is served, immediately push half of the meal aside to later be boxed up and taken home. If you expect to find the food too tempting, ask your server to box half of the meal when your food is served.

Dessert can be a fun part of any meal. Again, look at your choices. Are there some lower-calorie options like sorbet or fresh fruit? If you desire the double-rich chocolate cake, share one piece with your dinner companion(s) or box half of it and take it home for the next day.

Beverages can be challenging. Try to forgo the sodas and opt for water with lemon. Thus, you avoid empty calories. Consider sipping on sparkling water or mineral water throughout the meal, as it aids in digestion. If you'd like a mixed drink or a glass of wine, so be it. However, factor in these calories and sip slowly.

Remember, food and dining are meant to be pleasurable. Eat slowly, put your fork down between bites, chew methodically, and savor the tastes and textures of your food. Enjoy the company and the conversation. You are in control of your decisions.

HOW TO HANDLE FAMILY GATHERINGS AND PARTIES

An important tactic is not to go to family gatherings, parties, or restaurants when you haven't eaten all day. People often think that if they are planning to go out to eat, they should avoid food all day and thus "save up their calories" for the big feast. Unfortunately, this sets you up for failure. You arrive famished and are ready to eat anything and everything. You have also pushed your metabolism into "conservation mode," and it has begun to slow down. Eat fruits, vegetables, and protein throughout the day. You may want to keep your calorie intake a little lower to allow for the extra calories expected later. Stay on track with healthy eating and high-quality fuel for your body, and don't forget to exercise!

Family gatherings can be tough. There is often an abundance of food and drink everywhere! In some families, not eating what's served—and a lot of it—is considered offensive to the host. For many people, food implies love, and not eating that food sends the message that you are rejecting the cook's love for you. Carrying extra weight is the norm for some families. Why should you want to be any different? So, what do you do?

DEALING WITH OTHERS' REACTIONS TO YOUR WEIGHT LOSS

Making changes in your life may affect everyone around you in some form or another. These changes can even seem quite threatening to certain family members, friends, and co-workers, because they may subconsciously feel that *they* should be making changes to their own lives as well. Many people resist change and therefore want you to stay the same, too. You are a walking reminder that change for the better can occur and that one can reach a healthier weight. You are being successful, and they are not. They may resent this.

Hold your ground and keep in mind that you value yourself and are on the path to improved health. If it's too difficult and tempting to sit at the table after you finish eating, you may want to get up and offer to serve the coffee or begin to wash some dishes. You may want to enlist some family members who would like to go for a walk or start playing a board game. Try to occupy yourself and stay away from the food. These can be tough situations. If all else fails, you might need to leave the gathering early. This might be annoying to others, but you need to take care of yourself and stay on track.

Keep in mind, however, that if you "blow it," all is *not* lost. Do not revert to negative self-talk and dieting lingo. Do not tell yourself, "Well, why bother anymore? I've gone off of my diet, so what's the use?" Tomorrow is a new day, when you will get yourself right back on track. Eat in a healthy manner, lower the calorie count a little, and keep up your exercise. Remember, healthy living is a journey, not a race. Those little changes over time do add up!

Case Study: Kate

"I was able to get back on track."

Kate is a twenty-eight-year-old single mother with an eight-year-old son. She has a full-time job and a busy life. She first came to my clinic weighing 199 pounds. She was sixty-five inches tall, which put her BMI at thirty-four. Kate's cholesterol level was 230. Over three and a half months, Kate lost fifteen pounds and her cholesterol improved to 182. She has been able to eat a variety of foods, including chocolate, yet she has kept a food record and has maintained a 1450-calorie-per-day eating plan.

Kate did have a setback when she visited her relatives in a distant state. Much food was prepared for her, and she was expected to eat it! She tried not to let this upset her, and she made a choice to be particularly active. She took walks in the neighborhood, took her son to the zoo, and walked to the post office. She even cleaned her grandmother's house!

After her extended vacation, Kate came home and learned that she had gained six pounds. She had an afternoon of "panic," but then made the choice to get back on track. She did not give herself negative messages. She restarted her record keeping and weighed and measured her foods. Kate followed a 1350-calorie-per-day eating plan for the next two weeks and made sure that she walked 10,000 steps per day. By the time she came in to see me for her next visit, she had lost the six pounds previously gained and felt confident that she was back in control.

QUESTIONS TO ASK YOURSELF

1. What are the three main restaurants that I frequent?

2. What are some healthy choices that I can make at those restaurants?

3. Do I "starve" myself before eating out?

4. If I go overboard with my eating at a restaurant, party, or gathering, will I feel tempted to give up my quest to reach a healthier weight?

5. How does my family spend holidays with regards to eating and activity?

6. What three things can I do to stay on track this month?

MOVING FORWARD

1. You can make healthy choices at restaurants and parties.

2. Do not skip meals and "save" calories for an evening out.

3. Box half of your meal and take it home for lunch the next day.

4. Incorporate activity into your family gatherings.

5. If you go overboard with your eating, get back on track the next day.

6. Make smart choices about your food and calories.

7

I Don't Always Eat Because I'm Hungry

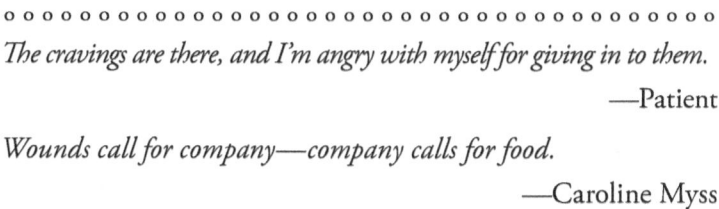

The cravings are there, and I'm angry with myself for giving in to them.

—Patient

Wounds call for company—company calls for food.

—Caroline Myss

EMOTIONAL AND PSYCHOLOGICAL FACTORS IN OVEREATING

Let's talk about this aspect of eating behavior. Many people eat when they aren't truly hungry, but rather stressed, lonely, anxious, upset, bored, or in emotional pain. Eating becomes a way of coping and self-medicating. They are often stuffing down not just the food, but their difficult feelings. Eating in this manner may provide some temporary relief, but it's also a way of avoiding serious underlying issues.

For example, one of my patients felt quite lonely in her marriage. She and her husband seemed to be leading parallel lives that didn't intersect. Instead of talking with him about her feelings and trying to deal with the marriage problems, she would sit in the kitchen and eat her "comfort foods" all evening, while he watched TV in the living room. Over the course of a year, she gained fifty pounds.

Comfort foods are often ones that contain simple carbohydrates. Foods like cookies, candy, cake, and pasta result in more tryptophan in the brain. Tryptophan is a precursor of the neurotransmitter serotonin—the "feel-good" chemical—which is why one temporarily feels relief from emotional pain when ingesting these foods. Eating comfort foods becomes a subconscious way of self-medicating. This type of eating also results in the release of brain endorphins and dopamine, both of which induce a greater "high" and sense of calm.

However, you must realize that these beneficial effects are very short-lived. Not long after ingesting comfort foods, feelings of shame, remorse, and self-loathing often occur. These negative feelings can lead to still more emotional overeating, and the extra calories will result in still more weight gain. So, what's a person to do? Are you doomed by this behavior forever? Not at all. Let's take a look at some possible solutions.

Before one can permanently change a behavior, one needs to understand why that behavior is occurring. What is triggering the feelings? What is triggering the eating? Many of us learned long ago to use food for comfort, reward, celebration, and even mourning. We have learned to eat when we're happy, when we're sad, and when we celebrate. How many of you went out for ice cream at the end of the school year to celebrate? How many of you were given food and drink to "help you feel better" when you were sad? How many of you associate going to the movies with buying popcorn? How many of you associate going to a baseball game with having hot dogs and beer? None of these things are "wrong." However, when you use food to avoid dealing with difficult issues and pain, patterns develop that can become self-destructive. Remember, these are *learned* behaviors that can *change*. You can develop the skills and the power to do so. It is in your control.

Begin by identifying why you may be participating in stress eating and mindless munching. Then, develop some strategies not involving food that will help you cope with your negative feelings in a healthier manner. For example, imagine that you've had a tough day at work. Somebody did something that hurt you, and it seems that you have no control over the situation. Instead of putting yourself down and binging on a package of cookies and a quart of ice cream, try to halt the negative self-talk by employing a healthier coping mechanism. These can include:

Taking a walk

Going for a swim

Dancing to some music

Taking a hot bath

Lifting weights

Writing in your journal

Playing with your pet

Planning a vacation

Checking your e-mail

Knitting

Woodworking

Gardening

Playing with your children

Talking with a friend, partner, or colleague

Developing a strategy for dealing with the difficult situation or person

One of my patients came up with a strategy that worked for her. In addition to emotional eating, she also liked to gamble. What she decided to do whenever boredom, unhappiness, anger, stress, or fatigue set in, triggering the desire to munch or gamble, was to put some larger clothes she had outgrown into a grocery bag, walk to the Goodwill store, and donate it. What a great idea! She got rid of her larger clothes, thus not giving herself permission to grow to that size again. She also got in some extra steps for the day and saved money too!

Another of my patients used to come home after a very stressful day at work and spend about thirty minutes in the kitchen eating higher-calorie snack foods to "relax." Before dinner, he would already have consumed over 1800 calories! He was able to change this habit by entering the house through the front door, thus avoiding the kitchen. He then changed into more comfortable clothing and went for a thirty-minute walk. This helped to reduce his stress levels, and he lost the desire to binge on junk foods.

The point is to do something more productive than eating to help you discharge the tension that has built up inside you. A helpful tool to increase your awareness of your emotional eating is to continue record keeping. In addition to logging your foods and activity for the day, you should also note your feelings and emotions. Then, you can go back and look for patterns between certain foods and feelings. When you are able to identify these patterns, you will become better able to make changes and healthier choices.

Table 7—Emotional Eating Record

Situation/event/ thoughts	Feelings/ emotions	Old coping strategy	New, healthy coping strategy
Late for work, boss glared at me	Annoyed and nervous	Drink two cups of coffee and have a doughnut	Drink a protein smoothie and do deep-breathing exercises
Had to run errands at lunch, got caught in traffic jam, another driver yelled at me	Pressured and angry	Yell back at rude driver, go to fast-food drive-thru, eat high-fat meal	Smile at other driver, order salad at drive-thru, use dressing and toppings sparingly
Shopped for groceries after work, bought more food than needed because I was hungry	Anxious and hurried	Purchase high-fat, high-calorie foods and convenience foods	Plan a weekly menu, shop when not time crunched, purchase healthier foods

It is hard to make a change. You might even need to ask yourself whether you truly *want* to change. Learning new behaviors takes time and practice. Think of all the methods I've suggested as individual baby steps. The first steps will be slow and halting. There will be falls. You'll keep trying, though. Before you know it, you'll be off and running with some healthier coping mechanisms, because you didn't give up.

The emotional aspects of eating can be very powerful, and some people might need to employ more tools to deal with this. Prescription medications can be helpful in modulating this type of behavior. These substances tweak various chemicals in the brain and in the gut to stabilize the overpowering drive to binge and self-medicate with food.

Many people with eating issues benefit by participating in individual or group therapy. This is a safe place to explore emotions that trigger unhealthy eating habits. Knowledge and acknowledgement are the first steps in taking back your self-control and establishing power over your eating habits.

SELF-ESTEEM AND WEIGHT GAIN (OR LOSS)

The greatest danger, that of losing one's own self, may pass off quietly as if it were nothing. Every other loss, that of an arm, a leg, five dollars, etc., is sure to be noticed.

—Søren Kierkegaard

Overweight and obese people attest to the fact that they are often "not noticed" and overlooked by others. In spite of obesity being a visible condition, the obese person can feel as though he is disappearing behind his own size. The subsequent loss of self-respect results in a devaluation of self. When you do not value yourself, you do not prioritize yourself and your needs.

One of my patients had lost and regained about a hundred pounds several times during her adult life. When she was diagnosed with diabetes type 2, she became quite alarmed, seeing it as a true wake-up call. She decided to take charge. She began to adhere to a healthy eating plan and started a daily walking program. She has been successful in losing weight and markedly improving her blood sugars. She told me at her most recent visit that she finally realized the need to "put myself first" and "take care of myself."

It takes time and planning to eat well and incorporate physical activity into your daily life. So many other aspects of daily life can seem to have more importance. Certainly, as one becomes heavier, feelings of shame and worthlessness increase, leading to more overeating. As one becomes heavier and the muscles get weaker, it becomes more difficult to move the body. It hurts. This perpetuates a vicious cycle of eating to self-medicate and "stuff down" negative feelings, which leads to further weight gain.

Challenge yourself to change this behavior by beginning to develop healthy habits that will lead to self-respect and inner strength. Begin with a plan. Commit to a ten-minute walk every day. Commit to one healthy food choice—only one—every day. You can do this, and when you accomplish it, your self-respect will grow. Before you know it, the ten-minute walk will have increased to a fifteen-minute walk, and then a twenty-minute walk. The one healthy food choice will have increased to two, and then three, and so forth.

By keeping this promise to yourself, you are acknowledging your self-worth, and your self-respect increases.

Another very powerful tool is "self-talk." In my practice, I am always amazed (and a bit saddened) when I hear a patient saying, "I've been bad," "I'm not good," or "I failed"—all because of a rough couple of weeks, a pound of weight gain, or the lack of weight loss. Why do we punish ourselves so much? Why do we feel the need to be perfect? Let go of the need for perfection. Negative talk serves to enhance feelings of low self-worth, which, in turn, can lead to more overeating, and then a further downward spiral of self-respect. It truly becomes a vicious cycle of self-sabotage.

Begin by reframing your thinking. Perhaps you haven't lost weight this week, but neither did you gain any, and that counts as a success! Yes, you had a doughnut for breakfast—but then you had a yogurt for your midmorning snack, and that was a healthy choice!

You may have gained a couple of pounds over the last month, but this doesn't make you "bad," nor are you a "failure." Why are you making a moral judgment about this? Try to think about why the weight gain has happened. Were you as active as you needed to be? Did you keep your food records? Was your mother in the hospital, the children sick, or the washing machine broken? Did you have to put in extra hours at work? There is a reason. Acknowledge it and the surrounding emotions, then keep going. This knowledge and understanding will give you increased control over the situation and the power and belief in yourself to continue to make positive choices. Next month will be better. Don't let life control you. Take charge! Try to prevent discouragement by:

Setting realistic goals	Nurturing yourself with positive self-talk
Making a list of five to ten things you like about yourself and reviewing it daily	Approaching your weight loss as a journey and not a quick fix
Eliminating "shoulds"	Decreasing your TV time
Not eating when watching TV	Being aware of your feelings and acknowledging them
Accepting that you are human and not perfect	Solving problems and making a plan
Asking for help	Rewarding yourself for reaching small goals

Realize that changing long-formed habits is difficult and that there will be bumps in the road. You are not perfect—no one is. What is important is that you continue the journey toward strength and health. Do not give up.

Case Study: Sophie

"I know I'm a binge eater."

Sophie came to see me when she was forty years old. She weighed 180 pounds and was five feet tall. Her BMI was thirty-six. Sophie had struggled for years with her weight and was ashamed of her body. In fact, initially, she wasn't even comfortable removing her jacket to allow me to take her blood pressure. She had been binging on food for years. She was on a roller coaster of binging that was invariably followed by shame and self-loathing.

Sophie was an accomplished attorney who kept her binging episodes secret from others. She told me that she was able to control her eating throughout the day. In fact, she was so busy that she didn't even eat that much at work. Breakfast was a latte. Lunch might have been a quick cup of soup—otherwise, she pretty much survived on coffee throughout the day. At the end of the day, though, she would go home stressed and anxious and use food for comfort. "I was starved!" she said.

Sophie had tried "every diet out there." She told me that she would usually be able to lose about fifteen pounds each time, but then she could no longer stand the restrictions and would go overboard. Sophie wasn't aware of when she was truly hungry or when she was truly full. I have now been seeing Sophie for two years. She has been able to lose thirty pounds and stay at 150 pounds for the last nine months. I've started her on appetite-suppressant medications, which have decreased her urge to binge. She has committed to eating breakfast, lunch, and an afternoon snack, so she is not overly hungry at the end of the day. She has also started a yoga class, which has helped reduce her stress.

At one point, Sophie shared with me that she had been raped in college, which she had never told anyone. She was able to admit that she was "hiding" behind her weight. She also realized that she was "stuffing down" the multitude of feelings that she had never dealt with. Sophie is now seeing a counselor every other week, and she checks in with me once a month. She is working on getting healthier—not only physically, but mentally and emotionally too. She has made and is making great strides. I am very proud of her!

QUESTIONS TO ASK YOURSELF

1. Do I eat to live, or do I live to eat?

2. What is the underlying motivation for my eating?

3. Do I listen to my body and pay attention to true hunger cues?

4. What are my trigger foods?

5. Who might be trying to sabotage my weight-loss efforts?

6. What makes it difficult for me to prioritize my needs?

7. What makes it difficult for me to feel positive about myself?

MOVING FORWARD

1. Make a list of five alternatives to eating that will help you deal with feelings of anger, loneliness, boredom, stress, and fatigue.

2. Consider participation in group or individual therapy.

3. Value yourself, regardless of your weight.

4. Remember that change takes time.

5. Embrace the positive changes you have made.

6. Realize that no one is perfect.

8

Is This the Right Time to Work on Weight Loss?

○ ○

If you choose not to decide, you still have made a choice.

—Neil Peart

Weight regulation is a complex issue and is the result of multiple interacting factors, so we need to try to address as many of these as possible. Healthy eating balanced with appropriate activity, use of medication (for some), lifestyle change, support systems, inner growth, and acceptance of self will result in a healthier and slimmer you—a person who is not defined by a number on a scale. I am not talking about you becoming model thin, but attaining a weight that is healthier for you.

When you begin a weight-loss journey, it is important to have realistic goals. What you weighed at twenty years of age most likely will not be what you will weigh at forty or fifty. Likewise, you must realize that the rate of loss should be slow and steady. Losing ten to twenty pounds per week is not safe, nor is it conducive to weight maintenance. This type of loss eventually has negative consequences on your body. Health issues associated with rapid weight loss can include dehydration, dry skin, hair loss, saggy and wrinkly skin, vitamin and mineral deficiencies, gallstone formation, loss of lean muscle mass, and a slowing of the metabolism that can make it difficult to reach a healthy weight in the future. Most importantly, rapid weight loss due to restrictive or extreme dieting *does not result in the maintenance of the new weight*.

Having unrealistic goals for weight loss can set one up for disappointment and failure. Here is an example. A forty-two-year-old woman at 5'4" tall weighs 218 pounds. Her lowest adult weight was 155 pounds, but she was able to maintain that for only three months. She has stated that her *dream* weight would be 125 pounds. She has said that she would be *happy* at 150 pounds, and she does agree that a weight of 164 pounds would be acceptable. She thinks that she would be very *unhappy* at a weight of 180 pounds. Realistically, even a weight loss of twenty pounds would improve her health and reduce her risk factors for disease. Reaching a weight of 125 pounds and being able to maintain it would not be very likely for her. I say this because this is a weight she has never reached as an adult—even the 155-pound level was difficult for her to maintain. Her body did not want to be there. So ponder these questions:

What is my dream weight?

At what weight would I be happy?

What is an acceptable weight for me?

At what weight would I be disappointed?

What is a weight that I can *realistically* maintain, given my schedule and lifestyle?

This last question is key. Would it be desirable to lose more than twenty pounds? Yes—most likely. But what kind of effort would that require? If it would mean you taking in 1200 calories a day and needing to exercise three hours a day indefinitely, how compatible would that be with your lifestyle and multiple responsibilities?

Reframe your thinking to focus on developing a healthy and fit body. Remember, we all come in different shapes and sizes. Reaching a healthier weight is attainable by portion control and moderate activity, which also allows you to fulfill your other life responsibilities. **Your ultimate goal should not be some specific number on a scale or a certain size of clothing**. Don't let the external define who you are as a person. You want to make sure that *you* are ready to address your weight issues and that you want to lose weight for the right reasons. Dig a little deeper, and ask yourself the following:

What is my motivation for losing weight?

How motivated am I right now to lose weight?

What purpose does being overweight serve for me?

What makes it difficult for me to take care of myself?

Why don't I care enough about myself to make my health a priority?

What are the positive aspects losing weight?

What are the negative aspects of losing weight?

How do I benefit from losing weight?

How certain am I that I can remain committed to a weight-loss program?

How do I feel about exercise?

How frequently do I exercise?

Am I willing to make changes in my lifestyle and day-to-day habits?

For example, a man who wants to lose weight in time for a class reunion, who really hates exercise, and who, deep down, is comfortable with being "invisible" due to being overweight, will probably not be as successful as someone who wants to lose weight to avoid diabetes, who can tolerate walking, and who has a goal of participating in a charity health walk. Your internal motivation will affect your success.

These are important questions to reflect on. Do some soul-searching. If you can answer these questions honestly and find that you are ready and willing to embark upon a weight-loss journey, let's begin! On the other hand, if you have a full-time career, three small children, an ill mother for whom you are caring, and church or volunteer commitments, this may not be the right time for you to take on the challenge of a significant lifestyle change. If you conclude that this isn't the right time for you, don't despair. Revisit the issue every two or three months. Take the plunge when it feels right for you. In the meantime, though, identify two or three habits that you might be able to modify relatively easily. For example, if you drink six sodas a day, cut back to three. If you don't usually eat breakfast, begin to do so. Commit to taking the stairs instead of the elevator. Even these small changes can result in some weight loss over time.

Instead of:	Choose:
Six sodas/day	Three sodas/day
No breakfast	Small breakfast (yogurt, protein shake, V8 juice, etc.)
Using the elevator	Using the stairs
Parking in a space close to the office	Parking at the outer edge of the parking lot
Eating lunch at your desk	Taking fifteen minutes of your lunch break and walking around the block
Hamburger and fries for lunch	Hamburger and apple slices for lunch
Cheese and crackers before dinner	Veggie tray before dinner
Ice cream while watching TV	Popcorn without butter while watching TV

Case Study: Annie

"My mind is now in the right place."

Annie is a forty-seven-year-old married mother of two very active boys. She also has a full-time career. She first came to my clinic a year ago weighing the most she had ever weighed—247 pounds. Annie is sixty-five inches tall, so her BMI was forty-three. She was very discouraged. The excessive weight was causing her to feel extremely tired, and she couldn't participate in activities that she used to enjoy like hiking, skiing, and waterskiing. Her joints were sore, her muscles ached, and her extra weight interfered with her ability to move. Annie had been on many different diets. Any weight she had ever lost, she had regained, and then some. Her family doctor had told her that she had developed early diabetes and sleep apnea and that she had to lose weight. Annie needed help.

Annie said that she wanted to get healthier. "My mind is now in the right place." Annie was ready. Over the course of the next year, Annie steadily lost weight. She did this by keeping a careful food record and gradually increasing her activity. Today, she is no longer record keeping, but is watching her intake and portion sizes. She reports that she and her treadmill "have developed a close working relationship." Even on busy days, Annie still makes time to exercise. She hasn't deviated from her plan for one year, in spite of vacations, holidays, and houseguests. As Annie puts it, "I need to do this for my health—and for me." In fourteen months, Annie has lost seventy-five pounds.

QUESTIONS TO ASK YOURSELF

1. Do I want to lose weight?

2. What is my weight-loss goal?

3. What is important to me about that number?

4. What is a realistic weight for me?

5. Am I ready to make some changes in my lifestyle?

MOVING FORWARD

1. Make sure you are ready to embark on a lifestyle change.

2. Be realistic about your goals.

3. Strive for a slow and steady weight loss.

9

This Is So Hard!

○ ○

The journey and not the arrival is what matters.

—T. S. Eliot

You have made the decision to lose weight, and *you can do it!* If you believe in yourself, you will be more likely to accomplish the task. Do not approach this from the perspective of dieting and restriction. A "diet" is something that you expect to end one day. Your lifestyle changes, on the other hand, can be permanent. Small, gradual changes that aren't too painful can result in slow and steady weight loss. Make a choice in favor of your own personal care and an investment in your health and well-being.

VIGILANCE, MAINTENANCE, AND ENCOURAGEMENT

Take small, incremental steps toward your overall goal. Today, you can choose to make some healthy food choices, and you can increase your activity. Tomorrow is another day. Remember, all of the desired changes will not take place overnight. You are learning new skills, just as you might once have learned to play the piano, ride a bike, swim, ski, make furniture, or create beautiful quilts. These activities took time to master—the same is true with lifestyle change.

Begin to think of food as fuel and energy for your body. There is no one *bad* food, as *all* food provides fuel and energy. In theory, you could lose weight if you ate nothing but chocolate chip cookies and candy bars, as long as you stayed within your daily calorie limits. This wouldn't necessarily be healthy, however, and you must remember that a variety of foods with varying tastes and textures will help you not feel deprived. If you go overboard one day, cut back the next day on your calorie intake and increase your calorie output. You have not "blown your diet."

Losing weight and keeping it off is an ongoing process. You will need to continue to be diligent about your food choices, and you will need to be physically active *always*. When you reach a healthy weight, you cannot stop the healthy habits that you have formed.

For those who struggle with weight regulation, diligence and vigilance must be lifelong. Regaining weight is associated with inconsistent and restrictive dieting, high stress levels, and emotional or binge-eating patterns. The good habits that you have developed have helped you to lose your weight. Now, you need to continue these habits to maintain your new weight. If you go back to your old ways, your old weight will come back as well.

Studies (Klem et al. 1997, 239–246) have examined people who have lost weight and maintained their new weight for as long as five years. All of these people shared certain characteristics. For example, they:

Ate breakfast

Continued to keep food records

Weighed themselves regularly

Exercised regularly—typically forty-five to sixty minutes per day, five to seven days per week

Had a good support system

Followed up regularly with their health-care providers for monitoring and support

Because weight regulation is an ongoing process and a challenge for many, most people do better with ongoing support and follow-up. Check in with your physician regularly, attend Weight Watchers or TOPS, and participate in a support group. Find the right balance for *you*. Set realistic goals and have the confidence and belief in yourself to reach them. Do not despair. Avoid crash diets and develop healthy habits. Remember, your goal is to have a fit and healthy body—not to reach some specific number on the scale! As one of my patients told me, "My weight does not reflect who I am inside."

THE SCALE

No one can make you feel inferior without your consent.
—Eleanor Roosevelt

Let me share with you a couple of thoughts about the scale and weigh-ins. I would encourage you to weigh yourself no more than once a week. Weight fluctuates from day to day, depending on fluid intake, activity levels, what you've eaten, and hormonal balance, among other things. It can be very discouraging to weigh yourself several times a day and see the number on the scale go up, down, and then up again!

Although it may seem to you that your excess weight was added almost overnight, it was not. Therefore, a slow and steady loss is advisable. This will happen as you begin to make those lifestyle changes we've discussed. Remember that muscle weighs more than fat. As you increase your exercise and develop more muscle mass, you may notice that the number on the scale does not move down—or even that it goes up a few pounds. This is normal. Don't panic! Keep on going forward. If you're taking in the right amount of calories in relation to what you're expending, your weight loss will continue.

Your weight-loss journey will see periods of weight loss, weight gain, and weight stagnation. At times, you will experience a steady decline in weight. Then, you might hit a plateau. The number on the scale may even go up a little, but, ultimately, it will go back down again. The *rate of loss over time* is what you should pay attention to.

Most importantly, do not let the number on the scale define who you are. Use it as a reality check. It can help you to be accountable to yourself, but don't let it divert you from your course. Your self-talk is important and powerful. It can either encourage or cause despair. Choose to encourage yourself and focus on positive changes, instead of verbally "beating yourself up" with negative messages. For example, should you step on the scale and see that your weight has increased by one pound, instead of berating yourself and stopping the positive behaviors you have developed, choose to remember that you have walked every day that week and that you have kept your food records for five days this week. You can also remind yourself that you've gone down one belt size. You tell yourself that this is a process, not a race. The following week, you will check your weight again, and you will stay the course. We all come in different shapes and sizes. Strive for a healthy weight and a fit body. Yes, the number on the scale is important, but so is your overall health and conditioning. Have confidence in yourself. You are a worthy person!

WEIGHT-LOSS GRAPH

START	0	1	2	3	4	5	6	7	8	9	10
	1										
	2										
	3	X									
P	4										
O	5		X								
U	6										
N	7										
D	8										
S	9			X							
	10				X						
	11										
	12										
L	13					X	X				
O	14										
S	15								X		
T	16										
	17							X			
	18										
	19									X	
	20										
	21										
	22										X
	23										
	24										
	25										

WEEKS

Figure 10
Sample Weight loss Graph

Case Study: Michael

"I was eating more than I realized."

Michael is a forty-five-year-old man who has struggled with his weight for many years. In high school, he played football and was a wrestler. At seventy-four inches tall and 250 pounds, he had been a big young man with a lot of muscle. Michael went on to play college football. However, as his life progressed, Michael's activity level decreased. He got married, established a full-time career, and had three children. He found little time for exercise. By the time he was forty-five, he weighed in at 340 pounds and had 32 percent body fat. Michael was increasingly tired and had developed sleep apnea and very high triglycerides.

Michael came to my office at the encouragement of his wife. He knew he had to make some changes, but it was hard! I assessed Michael's health, body composition, and RMR. I put him on a 2000-calorie-per-day eating plan and had him wear a pedometer. He was more than a little skeptical, but was willing to give my suggestions a chance.

When Michael started to track his eating, he realized how many calories he had been taking in. He was eating in the same manner as he had when he was an athlete in high school and college. However, he was now older, and his activity level had markedly declined. He realized that he was eating about 3500 calories per day, and not burning anywhere near enough of them.

Michael was motivated to change not only for his family's sake, but also for his own. He didn't feel well physically, nor did he feel good about himself. He began to plan his meals, made an effort to increase his steps, and even met with a counselor for about three months to deal with some deeper issues in his life.

Now, at the six-month mark, Michael has lost forty pounds and has committed to thirty minutes of increased activity each day. He has done this by restructuring his work schedule and going to the gym five days per week during his lunch hour. He has also stopped drinking two sodas a day and is eating three meals and an afternoon snack. He knows that he needs to continue to do this—at a minimum—for his health and well-being. It hasn't been easy for him, but he has stayed the course.

QUESTIONS TO ASK YOURSELF

1. What three things am I willing to change to achieve a healthier lifestyle?

2. How many days a week can I exercise?

3. Which days, and at what times?

4. How do I define a healthy and fit body?

MOVING FORWARD

1. Remember, this is not about dieting, but a manner of living.

2. Take small steps to reach your overall goal.

3. This is a *process*.

4. New habits need to be maintained.

5. Weigh yourself no more than once a week.

6. The number on the scale can be irrelevant.

10

Time to Pat Yourself on the Back!

Arriving at one goal is the starting point to another.

—John Dewey

It can be daunting, if not overwhelming, to focus on the need to lose fifty or a hundred pounds. When you give it a try and it doesn't happen overnight, there can be a great temptation to just say, "Forget it!" As we have discussed, although it may be necessary and ideal to lose a large amount of weight, it's better to break your overall goal into smaller increments. If fifty pounds is what you need to lose, begin with a goal of losing ten pounds. When you achieve this goal, set another of losing an additional ten pounds. Along the way, remember that you are focusing not on a number, but on health and fitness. Your ultimate goal is to develop healthy habits that will enable you not only to lose weight, but also to keep it off.

Changing a habit is difficult and takes time. This will not happen overnight. Don't beat yourself up—be patient with yourself! Likewise, when you reach your first goal, *celebrate!* It's extremely important to acknowledge your achievements and successes. You've worked hard, and you deserve to recognize your victories!

Reward yourself with something that is not food. For example, after a ten-pound loss, you could get a pedicure or buy yourself a new CD. When you've reached a twenty-pound loss, make the reward a little more significant. For example, buy a new piece of clothing. When you reach your overall goal of fifty pounds, do something special for yourself like buying a new pair of earrings, going away for the weekend with your spouse or a friend, or purchasing a new bicycle or a pair of good running shoes. Rewards don't need to be costly, but they should be meaningful to you. One of my patients, a full-time college student with two jobs, decided to reward her weight-loss accomplishment with nothing more complicated than an afternoon nap! *You* decide what will nurture you. What is right for one person might not be right for you. What is important is that you mark these milestones. You've earned it.

Likewise, if it took you a year to lose twenty pounds (and you want to realistically lose fifty), that's fine. You didn't *gain* twenty pounds, and you've made changes that are likely to be lifelong. You can now take the next year to lose another twenty pounds. Changing a habit that you've had for twenty or more years will not happen overnight. Psychologists have determined that it can take a person eighteen months to firmly cement a new habit into place! So be patient with yourself. People want quick fixes and easy solutions, but we all know that these ultimately don't exist. Persevere, and make those small and subtle changes that, in time, will result in further weight loss and the achievement of your healthy weight.

QUESTIONS TO ASK YOURSELF

1. How will I reward myself when I lose ten pounds?

2. How will I reward myself when I lose twenty-five pounds?

3. What five affirmations can I make about myself?

MOVING FORWARD

1. Take your weight-loss goal and break it down into segments.

2. Make small and gradual changes that you can maintain.

3. Reward yourself when you reach your milestones.

4. Persevere!

11

Moving Forward

QUESTIONS AND ANSWERS

Here are some questions that I often hear from my patients about food, exercise, medication, and results.

Food

How many grams of protein are there in chicken?

One ounce of meat, poultry, or seafood will give you seven grams of protein. So, for example, five ounces of grilled chicken provides thirty-five grams of protein.

How many grams of fat should I eat each day?

For a healthy heart and weight loss, I suggest that about 28 percent of your total calories be in the form of mono- or polyunsaturated fats. Each gram of fat is equal to nine calories. If your total calorie intake for the day is 1600, 450 calories should be from fat. This translates to fifty grams of fat per day.

Aren't nuts bad for you?

Remember, there is no one "bad" food. Nuts are an excellent source of protein, fiber, and essential fatty acids. However, because of their fat content, they are high in calories, so you should be conscious of your portion size.

What is the glycemic index?

The glycemic index is a scale that measures the amount of carbohydrates (sugars) in food. Foods with a higher glycemic index (GI) cause a sharp spike in glucose and insulin levels, and, over time, result in insulin resistance and toxic processes at the cellular level. This increased insulin resistance leads to weight gain. More weight gain leads to further insulin resistance, and thus, the cycle continues.

Why is it important to drink eight glasses of water per day when "dieting?"

Actually, whether one is working on weight loss or not, it is important to hydrate the body's tissues. If you are at all dehydrated (and this occurs before you ever sense thirst) the body's metabolism will slow down. This can result in a three-to-five-pound weight gain per year.

What are some good protein sources other than meat, chicken, and fish?

Protein is found in eggs, dairy products (like yogurt, cheese, and cottage cheese), nuts (including peanut butter), beans, and soy products.

I really like to have a glass of wine each evening. May I do this when I am working on weight loss?

Because you are not "dieting," feel free to enjoy your evening glass of wine. But make sure you take this into account when planning your eating for the day. Include the wine's 120 to 150 calories in your daily budget.

Isn't it best to eat three meals a day, and no more?

Actually, the body's metabolism functions much more efficiently and briskly when one eats four to six times per day. Spread your calories out over the course of the day by having breakfast, a midmorning snack, lunch, a mid-afternoon snack, dinner, and even a light evening snack. You will feel more satisfied and be less prone to binging and overeating.

Is it okay to have a doughnut for breakfast?

An occasional doughnut will not make or break your weight-loss plan. Having only a doughnut for breakfast, however, gives your body a rather high sugar load, which leads to a spike in your blood sugar, followed by a rather quick decline. This, in turn, triggers hunger. If you want the doughnut, have some yogurt or other protein source with it. This way, you are balancing out the sugar high with some protein, and you will feel a bit better sustained throughout the morning.

Exercise

How do I count my steps when I'm swimming and cannot wear my pedometer?

Assume that one minute of actual swimming (that is, doing actual laps and not just floating) equals 150 steps. Thus, a thirty-minute swim would give you 4500 steps.

I'm walking on the treadmill for twenty minutes at a time three times a week, but I'm not losing any more weight. I've reached a plateau after losing about twelve pounds. What should I do?

Congratulations on your twelve-pound weight loss! This is an achievement to be proud of. Now, if you want to lose more weight, you need to increase your activity. In addition, make sure that you're where you need to be with your calorie intake. Most people need to burn about 2100 exercise calories per week, at minimum, to lose weight. This averages to 300 exercise calories each day. Thus, you may want to walk five days per week instead of three and increase your time to thirty minutes each day. You could also add some light resistance training to your exercise regimen.

How many calories do you burn in walking one mile?

You burn approximately one hundred calories per mile. This estimate is based on a 154-pound male. If you weigh more, you burn more, and if you weigh less, you burn a little less. The amount also changes if you are a woman. However, for simplicity's sake, use the estimate of one hundred calories per mile.

I've heard that you shouldn't exercise at night. Is this true? What is the best exercise to do?

Exercising does increase your metabolic rate for a short period of time, even after you have finished exercising. Therefore, many people feel energized by exercising and may find it difficult to go to sleep immediately after an exercise session. This is why you may have heard that one should not exercise at night.

However, the best exercise is one that you enjoy and will continue to do, and the best time of day to exercise is whenever you will get it done!

I've gone down two pants sizes and am exercising more, but I've lost only twenty-four pounds. Why haven't I lost more weight?

Whenever you increase your exercise, there is a rebalancing period as you develop more muscle mass and lose fat mass. Muscle tissue weighs more than fat tissue. Thus, the number on the scale might not decrease significantly for a time, and it may even go up a pound or two. Yet, you've noticed that change in inches. You are developing a healthier body composition. As you progress and maintain consistent activity and calorie control, the number on the scale will again decrease!

Medication

I have high blood pressure and take medication to control it. Can I still use appetite-suppressant medications?

If your blood pressure is stable and under control, appetite suppressant medications usually do not present a problem. Of course, your blood pressure should be monitored regularly, and you should take these medications only under medical supervision.

I have had bariatric surgery. Do I need to take a protein supplement for the rest of my life?

The majority of people who have had gastric bypass surgery do need to supplement their diets with a protein shake or drink, usually once a day for the long term. This is because the stomach pouch is much smaller. There is also a component of malabsorption involved in this type of surgery. Therefore, it is difficult for most people to take in the required amount of protein through food alone.

Results

By the time I get home from work, I feel exhausted. After dinner, I usually sit in front of the TV and eat mindlessly. What should I do?

First of all, make sure to eat well throughout the day to prevent strong hunger and overeating when you get home. Make sure that you have adequate protein intake throughout the day, as this can maintain increased energy. If possible, try to get out of the office over the lunch hour for a walk, which will give you both physical exercise and a mental break. After dinner, even though you may feel tired and stressed, commit to thirty minutes of light walking, stretching, or yoga before sitting down to watch TV. The exercise can be invigorating and can break the desire to mindlessly eat.

I've had problems with infertility and am about eighty pounds overweight. One of my friends told me that if I lose weight, I might be able to get pregnant. Is this true?

Carrying excess weight is associated with (among other things) greater chances of infertility. The extra weight and associated insulin resistance affect the endocrine cycle and results in decreased ovulation. Even a loss of twenty-five to thirty pounds can result in a return to normal hormonal functioning and the improvement of an infertility condition. When working on weight loss, be sure to use adequate contraception if you do not wish to conceive, as fertility can return even with modest weight loss.

MOVING FORWARD

Reaching and maintaining a healthy weight doesn't have to be that difficult. Sure, it takes work, commitment, and a desire to make changes. It can happen, though, even as you continue to live your life, day to day. Small steps, even with some stumbles along the way, will get you to where you need to be. Believe in yourself, and never give up.

Here are some final tips for your journey into weight loss. Moving forward:

1. Make a vow to yourself to begin a healthy weight-loss program. Believe in your ability to succeed.

2. Have realistic and attainable goals.

3. Drink sixty-four or more ounces of water or unsweetened, non-caffeinated beverages per day.

4. Calories count! Be conscious of serving sizes.

5. Keep a journal and weigh and measure your foods, striving for 1400 calories per day for women and 1800 calories per day for men.

6. All foods are fair game, but try to stay within your calorie budget.

7. Strive for seventy to eighty grams of protein per day.

8. Do not skip meals.

9. Spread your calories throughout the day. Have breakfast, a midmorning snack, lunch, a midafternoon snack, and dinner.

10. Have nutritional balance at each meal.

11. Eat slowly, enjoying the flavors and textures of the food.

12. Chocolate can fit into a healthy eating plan.

13. Food labels can be misleading; read them carefully.

14. When eating at restaurants—where portions are often super-sized—ask your server to box half of your meal. Enjoy it the next day.

15. Desserts are okay.

16. Don't think of "dieting," but rather of eating in a way you can enjoy and maintain for the rest of your life

17. Practice moderation in all things.

18. Limit yourself to one pop per day. Or, better yet, drink none.

19. Think of food as fuel for your body—will it be high octane or low grade?

20. Buy a pedometer and strive to take 10,000 steps per day.

22. Take the stairs instead of the elevator.

23. Follow up with your doctor or participate regularly in a support system.

24. Celebrate your progress and milestones.

25. View this as a process, not a race.

Reader Resources

1. The American Society of Bariatric Physicians—www.asbp.org—A listing of bariatric physicians

2. The American Society of Bariatric Surgeons—www.asbs.org—A listing of bariatric surgeons

3. National Weight Control Registry—www.nwcr.ws—Information and research regarding successful weight maintenance

4. www.FitDay.com—Online record keeping

5. www.accusplit.com—A source for high-quality pedometers

6. www.CalorieKing.com—Online record keeping and a source for food and exercise journals

7. www.lapband.com—Information regarding lap banding

8. www.thedailyplate.com—Online record keeping

9. www.korr.com—Information regarding REEVUE

10. www.microlife.com—Information regarding the Body/Med Gem

Bibliography

Allison, D. B., Fontaine, K. R., Manson, J. E., Stevens, J., Van Itallie, T. B. (1999). Annual deaths attributable to obesity in the United States. *JAMA, 282*(16): 1530–1538.

Bays, Harold, Arbeeny, Cynthia. (2004). Obesity Pharmacotherapy: Perspective and Review. *Obesity Research, 12*(8), 1191, 1197.

Brownell, Kelly D., Wadden, Thomas A. (1999). *The LEARN Program for Weight Control.* Dallas, Texas: American Health Publishing Company.

Collins, J., Mattar, S., Qureshi, F., et al. (2007). Initial Outcomes of Laparoscopic Roux-en-Y Gastric Bypass in Morbidly Obese Adolescents. *Surgical Obesity Related Disorders 3*(2): 147–52.

Flegal, K. M., Carroll, M. D., Ogden, C. L., Johnson, C. L. (2002). Prevalence and trends in obesity among US adults. *JAMA,* 288: 1723–1727

Freedman, Marjorie R., King, Janet, and Kennedy, Eileen. (2001). Popular Diets: A scientific review. *Obesity Research, 9*, Supplement 1.

International Day for the Evaluation of Abdominal Obesity: Rationale and design of a primary care study on the prevalence of abdominal obesity and associated factors in 63 countries. (2005). *European Heart Journal Supplements*

Klem, M. L., Wing, R. R., McGuire, M. T.1997). A descriptive study of individuals successful at long-term maintenance of substantial weight loss. *American Journal of Clinical Nutrition, 66,* 239–246.

Knowler W. C., Barrett-Connor, E., Fowler, S. E.(2002). Diabetes Prevention Research Group. Reduction in the incidence of type 2 diabetes with lifestyle intervention or metformin. *New England Journal of Medicine 346*: 393–403.

Lichtman, S. W., Pisarka, K. (1992). Discrepancy between self-reported and actual caloric intake and exercise in obese subjects. *New England Journal of Medicine* 327:1893–1898.

Martin, Louis F. (2004). *Obesity Surgery.* New York: McGraw-Hill.

Mechanisms for metabolic dysregulation associated with obesity. (2006). *Obesity Research.* 14: Supplement 1.

Mokdad, Ali H., Marks, James S., Stroup, Donna F., Gerberding, Julie L. (2004). Actual causes of death in the United States, 2000. *Journal of the American Medical Association.* 291: 1238–1245.

National Consumer League obesity survey. (2007). *The Obesity Society Newsletter,* 5(7).

National Institute of Health, National Heart Blood Lung Institute. Obesity Education Initiative. (1998). Clinical Guidelines on the identification, evaluation, and treatment of overweight and obesity in adults. *Obesity Research,* 6(2), 51S–210S.

National Task Force on the Prevention and Treatment of Obesity. (2000). Overweight, obesity, and health risk. *Archives Internal Medicine, 160* 898–904.

Shape Up America! and the American Obesity Association. (1998–2001). *Guidance for Treatment of Adult Obesity.* Washington, D.C.: Shape Up America!.

Snyder, Eric, Brandon Walts, et al. (2004). The human obesity gene map: The 2003 update. *Obesity Research, 12*(3), 369.

Spiegel, Karine. (2004). Sleep curtailment in healthy young men is associated with decreased leptin levels, elevated ghrelin levels, and increased hunger and appetite. *Annals of Internal Medicine, 141,* 846–850, 885–886.

Sturm, Roland. (2002). UCLA/RAND Managed Care Center for Psychiatric Disorders. The effects of obesity, smoking, and drinking on medical problems and costs, *Health Affairs.* March/April.

Wansink, Brian. (2006). *Mindless Eating.* New York: Bantam Dell.

World Health Organization. (1998). Obesity: Preventing and managing the global epidemic. *Report of a WHO Consultation on Obesity.*

Endorsements

A unique, realistic, and motivational "journey" that truly inspires one to achieve and maintain a "healthy weigh." Dr. Baskett's medical and educational expertise shines forth! She is truly a master in clearly explaining the complexities involved in weight regulation. This book makes perfect sense.

Kathleen Renzi, MS
Program Consultant and Nutrition Educator
University of Maryland Cooperative Extension

"I have lost and kept off forty-two pounds over the last two years. Dr. Baskett has taught me how to manage my weight." —Patient

"I'm losing weight in the midst of living life. This plan really works!" —Patient

"This has been easy, and for once, I'm not on a diet." —Patient

"This is something I can do. Dr. Baskett's plan makes sense." —Patient

About the Author

Kathleen T. Baskett MD graduated from the University of Maryland School of Medicine. She became board certified in bariatric medicine in 1997 and is a Diplomate of the American Board of Bariatric Medicine.

Dr. Baskett is a member of the American Society of Bariatric Physicians and NAASO—The Obesity Society. She was the owner of the Montana Healthy Weight Management and Wellness Center in Missoula, Montana, and is the Medical Director of the St. Vincent Healthcare Weight Management Clinic in Billings, Montana. Dr. Baskett has published and lectured nationally on the topic of obesity. She has also participated in clinical research in the field of obesity. She has helped patients lose ten pounds, as well as 200+ pounds.

Dr. Baskett and her husband, Mark, live in Montana. Their children live in Hawaii, California, and Montana.